TOO YOUNG TO DIE

TOO YOUNG TO DIE:

The case for staying healthy and alive through preventive medicine

by

Donald R. Germann, M.D.

FARNSWORTH PUBLISHING COMPANY, INC.
Rockville Centre, New York 11570

All charts referred to in the text can be found in the Appendix (see pages 303 through 338). Charts VI, X and XXVII also appear in the text.

First printing.
Library of Congress Catalog Card No. 74-84337.
ISBN 0-87863-081-3.
Manufactured in the United States of America.

ACKNOWLEDGMENTS

Because the content of this book crosses virtually every specialty in medicine, massive research was involved both in gathering data and having all details checked by authorities wherever possible. I'm grateful to the many prominent physicians who gave of their valuable time to help assure the accuracy of the material and the conclusions drawn from it. Space prevents my detailing the contribution of each of these physicians so I will list them alphabetically and acknowledge that each made a significant contribution.

Allen, Max, M.D. Professor of Medicine
University of Kansas, Kansas City, Kans.
Ashenburg, N. S., M.D. Associate Medical Director
Eastman Kodak, Rochester, N.Y.
Athon, Merle, M.D. Family Practice
Overland Park, Kans.
Baeke, John, M.D. Family Practice
Overland Park, Kans.
Baylor, Curtis, M.D. Medical Director
Texaco, New York, N.Y.
Beeks, John, M.D. Industrial Physician
Ford Motor Company, Kansas City, Mo.
Berry, Max, M.D. Internist
Kansas City, Mo.
Blim, R. Don, M.D. Pediatrics
Kansas City, Mo.
Clemens, Al, M.D. Preferred Risk Insurance Co.
Des Moines, Iowa
Davis, Kieffer, M.D. Medical Director
Phillips Petroleum Co., Bartlesville, Okla.
Diamond, E. Grey, M.D. Cardiologist/Provost Univ. of Mo.
Kansas City School of Medicine, Kansas City, Mo.

Dodge, Mark, M.D. Internist
Kansas City, Mo.
Eberhart, C. M., M.D. Medical Director
Metropolitan Life Insurance Co., New York, N.Y.
Fowler, Fred, M.D. Neurosurgeon
Kansas City, Mo.
Gentry, Kale, M.D. Family Practice
Overland Park, Kans.
Gullett, C. C., M.D. Medical Director
TWA, Kansas City, Mo.
Hall, Ralph, M.D. Internist
Kansas City, Mo.
Hannas, R. R., Jr., M.D. Emergency Medicine
Evanston, Ill.
Hanson, Karl, M.D. Oncologist
Kansas City, Mo.
Hardy, John, M.D. Regional Physician
American Telephone and Telegraph, Kansas City, Mo.
Harless, Morris, M.D. Regional Medical Director
Montgomery Ward, Kansas City, Mo.
Hiebert, John, M.D. Cardiologist
Topeka, Kansas
Hunzicker, W. J., M.D. Medical Director
Kansas City Life Insurance Co., Kansas City, Mo.
Irving, Noble, M.D. Radiologist
Des Moines, Iowa
Kline, Edward, M.D. Cardiologist/Medical Director
General Electric, New York, N.Y.
Lauer, D. John, M.D. Chief Medical Director
International Telephone and Telegraph, New York, N.Y.
Lenci, A. D., M.D. Associate Medical Director
General Electric, New York, N.Y.
Levine, Edward J., M.D. Regional Medical Director
International Telephone and Telegraph, Chicago, Ill.
Levine, Harold, M.D. Chest Diseases
Hines Veterans Administration Hospital, Chicago, Ill.
MacGee, Edwin, M.D. Neurosurgeon
Kansas City, Mo.
Margo, Marvin, M.D. Orthopedist
Oklahoma City, Okla.
Mixon, William, M.D. Obstetrics and Gynecology
Kansas City, Mo.
Murphy, Franklin, M.D. Chairman of the Board
Times Mirror Corporation, Los Angeles, Calif.
Noback, Richard, M.D. Dean of the School of Medicine
University of Missouri at Kansas City, Kansas City, Mo.
Perry, Lawrence, M.D. Department Family Practice
University of Kansas, Kansas City, Kans.

Powell, Kenneth, M.D. Associate Medical Director
Kansas City Life Insurance Co., Kansas City, Mo.
Raich, Robert, M.D. Chest Diseases
Kansas City, Mo.
Roberts, G. G., M.D. Industrial Physician
Western Electric, Kansas City, Mo.
Serrano, J. R., M.D. Medical Director
Eastern Air Lines, Miami, Florida
Sutton, William, M.D. Medical Director
Eastman Kodak Company, Rochester, N.Y.
Van Ness, Lyle, M.D. Medical Director
State Farm Life Insurance Co., Bloomington, Ill.
Wescoe, W. Clarke, M.D. President
Sterling Drug Co., Inc., New York, N.Y.
Wheatley, George, M.D. Vice President and Chief Medical Director
Metropolitan Life Insurance Co., New York, N.Y.
White, George, M.D. Farm Bureau Life Insurance Co.,
Des Moines, Iowa
Wilber, Robert, M.D. Gastroenterologist
Kansas City, Mo.
Wynder, Ernest L. Epidemiologist/American Health Foundation
Editor "Preventive Medicine," New York, N.Y.

Not all assistance in preparing this manuscript came from physicians. I imposed on the patience and talents of many others. My needs were so great that local medical librarians would cringe when I entered.

My wife, a perfectionist housekeeper, permitted a section of the house to look like a disaster area as I read, wrote, discarded and rewrote this manuscript. Our hospital department typists had no free moments as they knew there were always extra letters or piece work to be done when regular work was finished.

Mr. Gene Murray, Assistant Editor of the "Star Magazine" was the first person I turned to for organizational and editorial help. I very much appreciate his hours and guidance.

Wanda Patton served as artistic consultant and general advisor throughout the entire creative period.

In the morale department—and every author must have periods when all looks hopeless, I want to thank my agent, Jack Dierks of Max Siegel and Associates of Chicago, Homer Wadsworth, now of the Cleveland Foundation, John Langley, Editor of University Press of Kansas and Tom Callear of Eastman Kodak. This book would never have been finished without their encouragement.

As I reflect on the help that was necessary to produce this book, it is amazing how many persons are involved. It is also very humbling to realize how many others have been needed.

Preface

One of the slogans used in the educational literature of the American Health Foundation states that "Nobody takes better care of you than you." Ability to take care of ourselves in health matters demands a knowledge of factors which lead to diseases and disabilities, as well as a knowledge of bodily functions in general. This book, well researched and written by Dr. Germann, serves both purposes. It describes the major causes of death in our population, what the known or suspected causative factors are, and how such factors can best be avoided. The book makes the point that, since many of our major diseases of today are man-made, it follows they are also preventable.

In order for these diseases to be preventable, however, it is necessary for the reader to realize that the message of this book applies to him or her personally. The book demands that the reader learn what risk factors are—for instance, blood pressure and serum cholesterol levels—and where and how to make the necessary adjustments. The fact that the individual should be in a position to demand preventive care from his or her physician is another constructive point the author makes in this book.

Dr. Germann correctly points out that preventive programs should begin in childhood, which is the time many chronic diseases originate. Parents ought to be obliged to read those chapters of the book dealing with the early lives of children. The resulting knowledge, when properly applied, could lead to a drastic reduction in both childhood and adult diseases.

The irony of preventive medicine is that it is a specialty which apparently provides no particular fascination for either physician or recipient. Preventive medicine is also faced with certain feelings of immortality which so many of us possess. The practice of good preventive medicine requires much self-discipline and it is this which Dr. Germann, and colleagues like him, find to be the greatest obstacle. Should the reader of this book come to the conclusion that he or she has a responsibility to maintain good health as a benefit to himself, his family, friends, co-workers, and to society in general, the lack of self-discipline common to all of us may yet be overcome.

Of course a book such as this can only present facts and offer advice. The impact, as usual, is up to the individual. It should be remembered, however, that throughout history none of our major diseases has ever been eliminated by curative medicine. Rather, it has always been preventive methods that have caused their elimination.

To paraphrase an ancient Greek adage, it should be the ultimate function of medicine "to help people die young as late as possible." If the readers of this book will follow its advice, this concept could become a reality.

—Ernest L. Wynder, M.D.

Dr. Wynder is president of the American Health Foundation and Editor of Preventive Medicine.

Table of Contents

Introduction

I graduated from medical school 25 years ago and spent the next six years in internship, residency, and military service. Fourteen years and a full professorship later, I abandoned academics for private practice in a large community hospital, where my specialty is diagnostic radiology and nuclear medicine. Both of these areas have an unending appetite for ideas and information and generate new tools and techniques that enable the physician to learn more about man and his diseases.

It has been an exciting 25 years. Today most neoplasms (cancers), vascular diseases, heart lesions, and degenerative diseases are both diagnosed and classified as to extent before treatment is undertaken. Therapeutic procedures have kept pace. Kidneys are transplanted, coronary circulation is reconstructed, and heart valves are replaced. These were only ideas a quarter of a century ago.

As one looks back, it is easy to lose perspective in the enthusiasm of accomplishment. We magnify our advances in the attempt to be more optimistic about the future. We also have a strange sense of values about life and publicity. We publicize our success in rebuilding coronary circulation, but we neglect to report that for every surgical repair several hundred people die of heart attacks. It seems strange that every death in a foreign political rebellion is reported individually by the news media, although we kill more people every weekend in the United States by automobile accidents than will die in that entire conflict. Each year more people die here of heart disease than have perished in all our foreign wars. While this does not justify political slaughter or war, it points up the fact that one death seems so much more important than another. Do we perhaps feel that war deaths are important because we believe they are preventable?

I hope that this is the reason, since the purpose of this book is to show that many of our most dread diseases are preventable and to demonstrate that death can, in many instances, be deferred. Your physician and I spend too much time and effort diagnosing hopeless disabilities or diseases with a 5 per cent survival rate. No matter how good our diagnosis or how successful our treatment, you would have been better off without the disease in the first place! Work with us. Let us make prevention of disease our goal for the last quarter of the 20th century.

This important work starts *now*. Ideally, your program should start at least one year prior to conception; if you are starting a family, your goals for your child require you to start planning immediately. Infants, children, and teenagers can improve their life expectancy more than we can estimate by starting now. Parental guidance is extremely important. If you are 30, 40, or 50, do not be discouraged by the first part of this paragraph. You are the most important of all to me. You are the productive people, and we need all hands producing at full capacity, at least until you reach the age of 65. We need to divide that ever-spiraling cost of government among as many productive people as possible in order to survive economically. Those over 65 are not forgotten, but the important habits required to defer death are best started early. However, better late in starting than not starting at all, for there is room for improvement if you start now. You can see that I have no intention of dying of any preventable disease. This makes my life expectancy about 100 years, and I need you to come along and share the taxes. We want to add years to your life and, even more, life to your years, so let us start *now*. Regardless of your age, you are *too young to die*.

Donald R. Germann, M. D.

I. The Facts of Death

Most people regard statistics as dull, and I agree. However, if we are to think in terms of preventing disease or delaying death, we should have a few facts about diseases and whom they select as their victims.

All good Americans complain about their government; I am no exception. When it comes to statistics, however, Washington is most productive. There are books, charts, and pamphlets for nearly everything that affects people. These are an invaluable source of material to me as a physician and author and to you as a consumer and critic. One encounters difficulty in acquiring very current statistics but, if we are willing to accept data as much as 5 to 6 years old, it is well organized and bound in book form. We will be dealing with large numbers, the trends of which we know, for we have many previous years for comparison. When more current information is available, it will be used, and other current sources will be quoted. I have been surprised to find many otherwise current books quoting statistics from 1960. (See in the Appendix, CHART XXVIII–*Mortality Trends for Ten-Year Period.*)

Chart I is taken from *Vital Statistics of the United States.* It lists in order, the 15 leading causes of death in this country. The rate is based on the number of deaths per 100,000 population. This chart is only a starting point, since we must adjust all of these causes of death for age. It will be no surprise to learn that there are no suicides under the age of six. It is also obvious that category 6, "Certain diseases of early infancy," is not a significant cause of death after the first year. It may be less well known that "Congenital malformations," category 13, produce death in all age groups. We also need to subdivide "Diseases of heart" and "Malignant neoplasms" for different age groups and different types of heart disease. Chart II resembles Chart I, but it is based on a 10 per cent sample of deaths in 1971. It is of value to demonstrate trends and offer more current data, but the detail we need cannot be accurately derived from it.

Chart III lists the death rate per 100,000 for each age group.

Several interesting observations can be drawn from these generally obvious facts. It seems that the most dangerous time of one's life is that at age less than one year. Of all one's life to age 80, the most dangerous time is day 1. It is also of interest that the safest time in one's life is from ages 5 to 15. However, the sharpest increase in risk comes between the groups aged 10 to 14 and 15 to 19. Of course, the very highest risk rate is that of those over 85. Such is the price of success.

Chart Number IV presents some very surprising data. I first encountered this chart in a book entitled *Physiology of Exercise* by Dr. Ernest Jokl. In his chart, the United States life expectancy curves were those of 1930. With the 1930 life expectancy data, the United States male life expectancy curve crossed the life expectancy curve of the Roman male at age 61. This seemed unbelievable to me. Therefore, I took the data from the *Vital Statistics* manual for 1967, and replotted it against the life expectancy curve of the ancient Roman, and found that the two curves now cross at approximately age 63. In making our own curve, my consultant physicist tended to smooth the Roman data; and because of this, the resulting two-year improvement in life expectancy may be more technical than real.

This chart offers many interesting points of speculation. We have been told repeatedly that there has been progressive improvement in life expectancy in this country. This is certainly true for the very young. A 1-year-old female child in this country has a life expectancy of nearly 76 years, which is an all-time high. The life expectancy of male infants is nearly 10 years less; throughout the entire spectrum of life expectancy, the male is at an obvious disadvantage until the 85th year. This was not the case in the Roman Empire. Males enjoyed the longer life expectancy. The female of age 15 could expect to live only 15 years longer. This was undoubtedly because of the high mortality that occurred with childbirth. It is noticeable that, as the Roman female approached the age of 40, her life expectancy improved slightly.

The most important concept that I can derive from this chart is that in 1967, as well as today, the male in the United States has no better life expectancy than the male of the Roman Empire, once he reaches age 60. To those of us in the medical field this is a shocking revelation. When I think of the extensive medical care that is delivered to patients in this age group, it is difficult to believe that statistical improvement has not occurred. We find and treat successfully many forms of malignant disease in people 60 years of age and older. The urologists save the elderly male who cannot pass urine because of prostatic obstruction. These people go on to live normal lives for many years; they would certainly have died in ancient times. Many of our patients in this age group have heart attacks, but survive. The elderly patient who falls and breaks a hip is surgically pinned and is usually up and able to move about in a relatively short period of time; even in my short period in medicine, this has been a dramatic improvement in the elderly patient. Antibiotics have made a great deal of difference in the outcome of infectious disease, not only in children, but also in patients over the age of 60. All of these facts make the revelations in the chart shocking.

Since we are quite certain that the medicine that is practiced today offers many benefits over that offered in the days of the Roman Empire, other factors must operate to counteract whatever positive effect the medical profession has been able to exert. These nonmedical influences are not too difficult to find. Modern man has acquired a new group of diseases; diseases once relatively rare have now become commonplace. Our Roman ancestor did not have the benefits of air pollution, cigarette smoking, a rich diet for an entire lifetime, high-speed automobiles, and alcoholic drinks that are much stronger than wine. As a result, he did not have the opportunity to develop our degree of arteriosclerosis, cancer of the lung, cirrhosis of the liver, and emphysema. Certainly, he suffered accidents in his charriot, but I doubt that they compared in seriousness with our automobile smash-ups. For these reasons, once our Roman ancestor reached the stage of life in which he was no longer a soldier in combat or driving recklessly in his charriot, his chances of enjoying a healthful elderly period were quite good. Our chart points out several other needs. The drop in life expectancy as demonstrated by the slope of the curves for both the American male and the female is steeper than we would like. The male curve could certainly be brought up to the female curve, although I fear that, as trends are beginning to develop, the female is beginning to drop toward the male curve. This may be one of the prices of the liberation of the American female. To improve these curves would seem a worthy goal.

II. Death Deferred

Everyone has some concept of preventive medicine. To most people it is the immunizations doctors give babies or the shots we must take when traveling overseas. Most people are also aware that sewage disposal, meat inspection, the work of the Food and Drug Administration, and a myriad of other similar, but less understood, functions have something to do with the health of the public. Each unit of government, from Washington to the local county, has public health offices involved in some of the many activities mentioned above. However, the term "death deferment" is meant to imply a more personal or individual activity that encompasses everything the government has to offer, everything you can get from your physician, and everything you can do for yourself.

No one will live forever. Just as the tax man will ultimately get his percentage of your deferred income, the grim reaper will someday be the winner. Our goal is not to live forever, but to live through those active, productive years in such good health that retirement will be an optional as well as an active, happy time. The death rate at all age groups is too high, but it is especially and unnecessarily high in the productive years between 35 and 65. Here death cheats society by felling vigorous, experienced, and talented people. In 1967 there were 1,851,323 deaths in this country, of which 715,161 occurred in people under the age of 65. This challenges us to reduce that number every year. There is no doubt in my mind that 100,000 deaths could be deferred immediately if the government, the physicians, and, above all, each individual would work toward that end.

The American public accepts preventive medicine quite well as long as it remains a passive process. By this I mean that the public in general accepts and promotes those activities that require minimal energy on the part of the individual. I have faith that this can be changed. The public certainly wants good sewage disposal, clean water, and clean air, and has offered only slight resistance to immunization programs.

Cooperation in cleaning up the environment is easy as long as it involves only other people. The public will bring tremendous pressure on industry to clean or eliminate the dirty smoke from its plants. Thanks to ecological pressure groups, all cars manufactured after 1976 will create little air contamination. But what about the older cars on the road now and at that time? No one has said much about making all car owners modify their cars to reduce emissions now or in the near future. I do not see why the car bought in 1976 as a new vehicle is so different from the car bought in 1973, but still in full operation in 1976. The most obvious difference seems to be that, by waiting until 1976 and then requiring these adjustments on new cars, we make industry responsible for the clean-up, since we assume they were responsible for all of the trouble in the first place. If old cars must be modified, who will do it? We might try to get the government to bear the expense, but it probably would refuse. We might even try to get the manufacturers to recall all older models for modifications, but they certainly would not do so. So it would appear that, if the older car is to be modified, it will have to be done at the expense of the owner. So, 1976 became the starting time.

So it is in the field of preventive medicine. We are pleased that the government insists on clean drinking water and enforces quality controls on most of the food we consume. We will even take, with only moderate reluctance, shots to insure ourselves and the public against disease. However, we do a much poorer job when health insurance requires active participation by each individual. Over the years our government has spent billions of dollars on medical research. Much of this has paid off; polio vaccine is the classic example. In fact, research expenditures have all paid dividends in one way or another. Many things we have learned have not proved popular, however.

For example, despite the billions spent on cancer research, we have found no cure-all and no overall preventive for that disease. We have learned a great deal about cancer; we know that in some instances it can be cured. We know that chemicals and irritants produce some forms of it. The surest thing we have learned is that tobacco is one of the most common, widespread carcinogens in existence. The popularity of this concept is evident in the ever-increasing cigarette sales. There is no doubt that what the public wants from the medical research man is an easy preventive measure for cancer, heart disease, and stroke. He would like to be immunized as a child and then no longer worry about these dread diseases. If that is a bit too much for physicians to produce in the next year or two, he would accept, as successful research, a pill that would cure these diseases once they occurred. Alternatively, with a flair for the dramatic, he would even accept an operation, with a long ugly scar to show his friends, as successful research if he were assured a cure and minimal inconvenience.

Without spending another nickel on research we could easily defer 100,000 deaths per year in people under the age of 65 if we would but practice the well-established disease and accident preventives already known to us. Let me list them here; we will elaborate on them as this book progresses. They are not necessarily given in order of importance.

1. Use seat belts and other safety devices in autos for adults and children.

2. Reduce alcohol consumption, for auto drivers especially, but for everyone in general.

3. Reduce tobacco consumption, especially cigarettes.

4. Control obesity.

5. Reduce the amount of cholesterol and saturated fats in all diets.

6. Institute an active exercise program for all ages.

7. Have regular physical examinations. Follow your physician's advice on how frequently this should be done in your case. If unexplained symptoms arise, see or speak to him about them at any time.

8. Cultivate an awareness of home accidents and poisoning. Establish a program within your household to prevent them.

9. Utilize prenatal care or, more important, preconception health care. This may become the hottest subject in medicine in the next ten years. It will make important strides in reducing infant mortality.

10. Cultivate knowledge and understanding of your physical and mental abilities and limitations and make constant efforts toward improvement.

This is an unfortunate list in the sense that every item requires action on the part of the individual. The government can insist on seat belts, but you must fasten them. The government can warn you about cigarettes, but you must quit smoking. Your doctor can tell you to exercise, but you must do it. Your father images (the government, your doctor, and industry) can lead you by the hand only so far. After that, it is up to you. The rest of this book will be spent showing you why and how very important these preventive measures are. If you want a long and vigorous life, you have an excellent opportunity to achieve it. Even more important, you can help give it to generations to come—if you are interested. It is my responsibility to motivate you to the point that you are willing to examine your life style and make important changes.

III. Health:
Define, Measure, and Keep It

When one attempts to define health, many different concepts come to mind. One dictionary defines it as "soundness of the organism." Fitness, soundness, vigor, happiness, enthusiasm—all of these words are used as synonyms of health. However, not one of them conveys the completeness that the word health seems to encompass.

Health certainly means different things to different people. To the octogenarian, good health means simply the ability to take care of oneself. To the new mother health may be synonymous with a vigorous cry and lusty appetite. To most physicians good health is simply the absence of disease.

The physician's assumption that health is no more than the absence of disease is most unfortunate. It is nevertheless an understandable fact. Since physicians are called primarily to diagnose and treat disease, they have only a limited opportunity to prescribe health. Certainly, when we think of the tools of medicine in terms of quantifying health, they are grossly inadequate. All too frequently a patient goes to his physician for a checkup, is pronounced to be in good health, and dies shortly thereafter of a heart attack. Dr. Lewis Kuller of Baltimore reported on a series of sudden-death patients in *The American Journal of Cardiology* for November 1969. He found that 23 per cent of sudden-death heart attack victims had seen their doctor within one week and that only 8.4 per cent had not seen a physician within one month. This is important information. It implies that the victim had a sense of impending disaster or something less; still, he consulted his doctor, and no definite diagnosis was established, or at least no corrective measures could be made effective. This sequence of events does not mean that the doctor was inept. It means only that most physicians are trained in matters of disease and its treatment and have limited abilities and tools with which to diagnose events of the future or to quantify this nebulous entity we refer to as good health. *This makes it very, very important that you learn how to keep from getting in trouble. This is what we mean by preventive medicine.*

Of all physicians, the pediatrician has a tremendous advantage over others in the matter of evaluating health. By virtue of his specialty, he is highly involved in preventive medicine. He is also involved in the development of good health habits, particularly in matters of nutrition and general guidance to his young patient. The healthy pediatric patient grows and develops. Therefore, the pediatrician who measures the height and weight of his patient with each visit and checks his intellectual and mental proggess has an ideal way of evaluating the health status of the youngster. If growth and development are normal for the first two years of life and then suddenly change, the pediatrician is immediately alerted that something has happened. Either the child has acquired disease, or the child's health has been altered in some other way. Unfortunately, when growth is completed, no such maneuver is available to the observing physician.

As a radiologist, I can speak with some authority and certainly most critically of the X ray and its role in evaluating patients in their states of disease and health. The chest X ray is a remarkable tool. From it we can establish very important information regarding the diagnosis and the stage of disease and even acquire a reasonable idea of its outcome or prognosis. However, if there is no disease to be identified, one must conclude that the chest is normal. We can make no statements in regard to the ability of this patient's heart to respond to stress or his lungs to exchange air. We can say only that this patient has the fundamental tools and that these tools are free of gross disease. Therefore, he should be able to function as a normal individual. As physicians, we know that any person sitting in an easy chair reading a book or watching television will normally not be short of breath. We know that to survive and supply adequate oxygenation of blood under sedentary conditions requires only about 15 per cent of one's normal lung capacity. Therefore, if we use as normal the absence of shortness of breath at rest, everyone with at least 15 per cent of lung function would be normal. On the other hand, if one runs up several flights of stairs, the demand on one's heart and lungs changes immeasurably. The chest X ray offers very little real information for determining if this patient gets short of breath while at rest or if he may be short of breath only after running up several flights of stairs.

The heart, which is so clearly outlined in the chest film, is likewise poorly evaluated in terms of its functional activity. There is no doubt that the chest film can identify certain valve lesions of the heart. It also tells us when the heart is too large or even when it is failing. Here again, there is no way of telling how the heart will react to stress. Certainly, the chest X ray would be the poorest criterion to use if one were trying to predict whether a patient would have a heart attack in the forseeable future.

Pulmonary emphysema, a very severe disease of the lungs, is in its early stages very difficult to identify radiologically. In its later stages, overinflation of the lungs and the appearance of poor tone make for ready diagnosis. However, by this time the patient becomes short of breath after a slight amount of exercise. If we are to make this diagnosis early, other tests such as that for vital capacity (measure of the volume of air expired from the lung after deep inspiration) will be needed.

One could go on with many other examples. An X ray of the skull certainly gives no evidence of the patient's intelligence or his personality. The X ray of the skull, however, may be extremely valuable in the identification of brain tumors, skull injuries, or even some degenerative processes.

I have used the X ray as an example of the medical profession's inability to measure health, but certainly the laboratory, the EKG, the history, and the physical examination all are geared for the diagnosis and identification of disease rather than the quantification and classification of health. Freedom from disease is indeed a very important aspect of health. Before one can be declared healthy or before any attempt is made to establish the degree of health, one must absolutely be free of disease.

The electrocardiogram is a most respected instrument in evaluating the cardiac status of patients. The electrical conduction system of the heart is altered by areas of heart damage; the electrocardiogram detects these changes. Once again we are detecting changes that occur after the fact. The extent of the disease may be determined by the electrocardiogram; if the recording is performed with the patient under stress, it may detect areas of disease small enough to be relatively asymptomatic. It is in this way that a small area of abnormality is detected and located so that other studies may be carried out. In order to bring out these minor changes, the electrocardiogram must be performed with the patient exercising or immediately following exercise. If the electrocardiogram is normal under these stressful situations, we have every reason to believe that the circulation or the coronary blood supply to the heart is adequate. In this way again, by ruling out disease, the electrocardiogram can be of value in measuring health.

The laboratory can be a valuable aid in the physician's attempt to evaluate the health of patients. Certainly, it is invaluable in determining the presence of disease states. There are some diseases that produce few or no symptoms and depend upon the laboratory for their detection. Such diseases include diabetes and early forms of liver and kidney disease. Blood determinations of cholesterol and fatty acids may give an indication as to the metabolic processes of patients and offer some warning as to the development of arteriosclerosis or coronary heart disease. Therefore, the laboratory, which the physician may use in varying degrees, is very helpful in identifying disease even if that disease is asymptomatic. Hopefully, the laboratory offers some quantitative evidence of health and disease prevention.

The history of the patient and the physical examination are very important in evaluation of health, but probably less important than they are in the diagnosis of disease. These serve as the physician's greatest asset to diagnosis and treatment. Of all diseases diagnosed, some 75 per cent are diagnosable from the history and physical examination. The laboratory and X ray findings serve primarily for their confirmation.

Medical histories are notoriously disease-oriented. Probing questions are asked in an attempt to find symptoms. When symptoms are expressed, other questions are asked in an attempt to elaborate on these findings. Poor health habits may be pointed out, dietary improprieties are noted, and corrective measures are offered as part of a summary to the patient. The physical examination is also disease-search oriented. The primary purpose of the physical examination is to observe and record findings. Very significant asymptomatic lesions may be found by this means. It is a very valuable procedure.

If the history, physical examination, X ray, laboratory tests, and electrocardiogram all fail to reveal any significant disease, the patient is said to be in good health. As we have said before, this is not necessarily true. We are simply stating that the patient is free of disease insofar as we are able to determine. One might well ask the question, "How good is my health?" To this question virtually all physicians would have a very limited answer. Since health also includes mental health and one's emotional attitudes, the physician is extremely limited in offering quantitative answers to your questions. Perhaps these questions are best asked by and answered by you. Your physician will find these questions helpful, but you must determine the answers.

1. Probably the most important of all—What is your resting pulse rate? Have your wife or husband take your pulse when you are asleep or take it yourself when completely relaxed and comfortable. This is one of the most critical measurements of heart function. We will strive to improve it.

2. How far can you run, walk, or combine running and walking in 12 minutes? This is Dr. Kenneth Cooper's physical fitness test. It is a vigorous quantitive test of heart, lungs, and musculoskeletal function. This is a real quantitive measure of health.

3. How many days' work did you miss last year because of illness? This is a quantitive question that not only covers your physical health, but gives some idea about how you feel toward your job.

4. How many books have you read in the past six months? This is a quantitive question to evaluate the vigor of your intellectual appetite.

5. What is your monthly expenditure in dollars and cents for sedatives, pain relievers, alcohol, and tobacco? Again a quantitive question designed to evaluate your physical complaints, mental anxieties, and bad habits.

There are undoubtedly other questions that would be important in the quantification of health. However, since quantitating health is a new experience to most of us, these initial questions certainly offer more information than we have used in the past. It is hoped that additional pertinent questions will be added by others interested in health. It is important that each of you answer these questions very honestly and record the answers. Questions 1, 2, and 5 should be evaluated on a monthly basis. Questions 3 and 4 can be answered only on a semiannual basis.

Now let me reply to each of the five questions as I think they would be answered by the average American male between the ages of 35 and 55. We all understand that there is no such individual as the average American male; therefore, your answers will probably be different for each specific question. Let us assume that this male has just completed a visit to his physician, where he went through a good routine physical checkup. In his final discussion with his physician he was told that there was no evidence of disease. He was a little overweight. He was told he should start some type of regular exercise and that he should stop smoking. The details given by the physician on how each of these steps were to be accomplished were quite specific in some areas. Since we are discussing an average American patient, we must assume that the advice received was from an average American physician. As our average American patient looked across the desk at our average American physician, he saw a man who was also a little overweight, a man who appeared somewhat tired. There may even have been an ashtray on his desk. So our patient was told that he was free of disease and in this the patient was truly reassured. However, when he evaluated the rest of the advice he was given, there may well have been a credibility gap. The physician himself probably needed a diet regime and an exercise program, but he offered no specific plan to our patient.

Question I. What is your resting pulse rate? There are diseases in virtually all age groups that result in a very rapid resting pulse. There are also some diseases, usually in the elderly, that result in a very slow pulse. However, since our patient has just been to the physician and is free of disease, we want his pulse rate to be in the normal range. We assume it is. The normal pulse rate range is relatively wide, but there are some pulse rates that are better than others. Here we start to evaluate your physical conditioning. Most physicians would accept a pulse rate from 50 to 90 as normal for the age group we have indicated. The American Heart Association lists normal as 50 to 100. However, I can assure you I would much rather have a resting pulse rate of 50 than 90, and one of the goals of your health program will be to get that resting pulse rate down. If you are truly well rested or asleep when the pulse is taken, and if that pulse is in the 80s, you have a lot of work to do. Our goal will be to keep it in the low 60s or upper 50s. Our average American patient is much more inclined to be in the pulse rate range of the high 70s or 80s than he is in the 50s or 60s. In order to lower the pulse, he will need to lose the excessive weight and establish a real physical conditioning program. (Score 0 for 65, +1 for each beat per minute less than 65, and –1 for each beat per minute over 65.)

Question II. How far can you propel yourself in 12 minutes? This question is in a way related to the first. However, it implies involvement of the lungs and the musculoskeletal system, as well as the heart. Most of us can walk a mile in 16 minutes with relative ease. A little extra jogging in the course of the mile should reduce the time to 12 minutes. Even though our patient just passed his physical, this test should initially be more walking than running. As our patient loses his few additional pounds and as his muscle tone, particularly his heart muscle, improves, he will gradually find that he can go farther and farther in the 12-minute test period. For our indicated age group we would like to see him get to a mile and a half for 12 minutes, possibly better. As this distance increases, you will truly have a quantitative measure of your improving health. (Score 0 for 1.25 miles, +5 for each .1 mile over 1.25 and –3 for each .1 mile less than 1.25.)

Question III. How many days' work did you miss last year because of illness? Since we are discussing the average American, we can give a much better answer to this question than we can to any of the others. A survey conducted by the American Medical Association and the National Center for Health Statistics gives us some very specific figures on the average amount of time missed from work by each employee. It varies somewhat with the region of the country in which our average American resides; however, 16 days missed from work for illness seems to be a reliable figure. It is also of interest to note that the employee making $15,000 per year or more averaged only 11 days of lost work each year, while the employee making $3000 or less per year missed an average of 29.3 days for disability. This is just another example of the tremendous cost of illness to this nation. (Score 0 for 16 days of absence in one year, +1 for each day less than 16, and –1 for each day more than 16.)

Question IV. How many books have you read in the past six months? This is probably an unfair question. I am sure many intellectually active people have read one or none. Certainly, our average American patient reads less than one book per year. However, an active reading program should be encouraged. After all, we are going to increase the efficiency of our heart and skeletal system by using them. The same is true of our intellect. There is no way in which it can be stimulated to produce and improve except by vigorous use. Therefore, our suggestion is that you increase from that less than one book per year to at least three. Once you start, this will be no problem. Each book will tend to stimulate the need and desire for others, and you will develop a self-perpetuating improvement program. The most difficult one is the first; since you are already started, I hope some of the references that we give will serve to make the next selection easy. (Score 0 for 3, –4 for each less than 3, and +2 for each over 3.)

Question V. What is your monthly expenditure in dollars and cents for sedatives, pain relievers, alcohol, and tobacco? Certainly, one's finances are purely a personal matter. I hope that you will sit down and try to calculate the dollars and cents you expend in this way. As the answers to the previous questions all improve, there is no doubt that the dollar figure for number 5 will decrease. I am sure that there are many people in the country for whom this value will be in the range of $100.00 per month or more. At this point we shall not incriminate the health role of any one of these four entries, but there can be no question that there is an adverse relationship of their usage to patient health. Therefore, as one's physical and mental health betters, there seems to be little doubt that one's financial health will also improve. (Score 0 for $10, +2 for each dollar less than $10, and –2 for each dollar greater than $10.)

Now add up your score. If you fit our criteria, you end up with a total of 0. If you have a minus number, you have work to do. If you have a plus number, you still have work to do. We all need to improve.

IV. Population Problems

We intend to show you how at least 100,000 deaths each year can be avoided with a moderate amount of personal discipline. Before proceeding with further details of this project, I am going to devote a moderate amount of space to the population problem. Reducing infant mortality rate or deferring death of the young and productive does not automatically have an associated increase in the earth's resources! I do not feel that a physician should apologize for attempting to improve life, whether qualitatively or quantitatively. However, to make no comments in reference to the population problem would be to imply that it does not exist, and no intelligent person would deny that world population growth is a problem. Hope is being offered to defer death, which does compound the population problem. At the same time other suggestions will be made that will slow the population growth rate. Hopefully, the total picture will be one of an improved quality of life without making the additional quantity burdensome.

In 1968 Dr. Paul Ehrlich published a very popular book entitled *The Population Bomb.* This one book has done more to interest people in the problem of overpopulation than any single publication in our time. Dr. Ehrlich presents the problem of overpopulation very graphically and substantiates his impressions with significant data. He has been accused of overstating and overemphasizing the problem;

however, any teacher knows that this is one of the finest ways to make a point. Certainly, Dr. Ehrlich has made a strong point, and that point is simply that there are too many people in the world.

Population growth rates are extremely important. It is on this basis that we can estimate the time required for a given population to double its numbers. The percentage of increase tends to be higher in the underdeveloped countries and lower in the more developed nations. However, if we are to consider the world as a whole, the following information from the United Nations is pertinent. It reports that in 1970 the world population reached 3,633,000,000 people. The average birth rate throughout the world was 34 per 1000, and the average death rate was 14 per 1000, giving a constant 2 per cent annual increase in the population. A 2 per cent growth rate results in a population doubling time of 34.6 years. This frightening figure suggests that, only a few years after we reach the year 2000, we will have 7 billion inhabitants. The highest population growth rates have been registered in some of the South American and Latin American countries, where they have been as high at 3.4 per cent per year. The European countries and the United States account for approximately 1 per cent increase per year.

Let us evaluate the year of interest, 1967. The following figures are readily available from the vital statistics of that year*:

	1967	1971
Births	3,520,959	3,560,000
Deaths	1,851,323	1,921,000
Net Increase	1,669,636	1,639,000

*Estimates of births and deaths for 1971 have been obtained from Editor of *Statistical Bulletin of Metropolitan Life Insurance Company*. They are presented for more current interest, but are not as accurate as those for 1967.

The population of the United States in 1967 was slightly below 200 million; however, this is a convenient number mathematically, and by using it we determine that the increase in our population was 0.835 per cent.

Now let us repeat the above subtraction problem using 100,000 fewer deaths and see what this does to our population growth:

3,520,959	Births
−1,751,323	Deaths
1,769,636	Net Increase

Based on these figures, the population growth rate is .885 per cent. Since we have already stated that the doubling time is extremely important, we can evaluate these percentage increases on that basis. We find that with .835 per cent, our doubling time is 83.5 years, while with .885 per cent the doubling time drops to 78.3 years. As we can see from this bit of arithmetic, 100,000 fewer deaths per year alters the population picture to a moderate degree.

The working force of any given population is considered to comprise those between the ages of 15 and 64. That percentage of the total population must support the entire group. The percentage of the total population represented by this group varies from country to country. In the United States approximately 60 per cent of the people are between the ages of 15 and 64. We are well aware that all people in this age group are not actively working and productive. Some are still in school. Others become ill. The President's Commission on Heart Disease, Cancer, and Stroke reported that the economic loss to this nation by direct and indirect means because of illness is in the area of $32 billion per year. Therefore, any possible illness or accident-prevention measures could be reflected significantly in the economic welfare of our country. In addition to this obvious saving, one of the finest contributions we might make to our total population program would be to return the dependent nonworkers, particularly those over 65, to the productive force in our population. By the maintenance of good health, a man could easily be productive into his seventh or possibly his eighth decade. By doing so, this man no longer would be living by the efforts of others, but would be supporting himself and helping to support the large dependent portion of the population. This would be good for the population as a whole and also immensely profitable to the individual. It should be our ambitious goal to have a high percentage of the population self-sustaining. It also seems logical that a larger number of people can enjoy a better life if we are not called on to support thousands of cases of preventable sickness and disability. Even though population growth remains one of the world's most serious problems, certain internal rearrangements will tend to negate the effect of the staggering population growth.

As one looks at the chart of birth rates over the past several years, it is apparent that our birth rate is falling. This decline in the birth rate started in the late 1950's, when it was nearly 25 per 1000, to the very recently reported birth rate of 15.8 per 1000 in the first quarter of 1972. This birth rate is the lowest recorded rate in our history. Remember, however, that there were a large number of babies born in the late forties and early fifties. The birth rate per thousand may be down, but there are many thousands in the child bearing age.* The only dependable calculation of population growth deals with the actual number of births minus the number of deaths divided by the total population, as we did it earlier. Wait until the end of the year and get the true numbers. In the year of our particular interest in this text, 1967, the birth rate was 17.8. In 1970, the birth

*Current estimate of babies born in 1972 is 3,256,000. This is the smallest number of babies born in any one year since 1946; note, however, that it is less than 1 percent under 1967. Deaths for 1972 are not available.

rate did jump to 18.3 per thousand, and at this point there was concern as to a renewed increased birth rate cycle. The latest figures I have quoted are reassuring in this regard. The lowered birth rate is at least in part a reflection of the increased number of abortions occurring in this country. We know that the current legal abortion rate is approximately 30,000 per month. This must have a significant effect on the birth rate. In this sense, abortion contributes to the solution of the population problem. However, in the same sense, so do war, heart disease, stroke, and many other illnesses. It would seem that more scientific indications for abortion might be more profitable than its indiscriminate use. There is no doubt in my mind that the birth rate can be significantly lowered if parents are educated to the proposition that they should emphasize quality in infants rather than quantity.

Dr. Paul Ehrlich is not the only authority in the field of demography, the scientific study of population statistics. One of the more interesting books on the subject is entitled *The American Population Debate.* Edited by Daniel Callahan, it is made up of a series of essays by 23 authors. One of these authors is Dr. Ehrlich himself. Another, who tends to oppose Dr. Ehrlich's views, is Ben Wattenberg; his essay is entitled "The Nonsense Explosion." Mr. Wattenberg is very encouraging as he points out that crises do not develop overnight in a world that is a billion years old. He emphasizes our falling birth rate, which has existed for nearly 20 years, and he feels that, even with a population growth of zero, many of our ecological problems will remain. Still, as one reads the many essayists in this field of vital importance, one cannot help feeling that there is a problem of too many people, too many pets, too many cars, too much leisure, and perhaps more important, too much careless consumption of our resources on the part of each of us as individuals. All of these things combine to result in shortages of food, goods and, of immediate interest, energy.

Despite the population problems, since I feel that productive people are worth more than sick people, I have no problem of conscience when I offer the opportunity of decreasing our deaths by 100,000 people per year. I am a physician, and my basic discipline is the avoidance of death and illness.

My offer is one of self-preservation. I hope to guide you in such a way that you can escape being a mortality figure during the tremendously important productive years. In so doing, you will avoid illness in general and generate health of such a quality that it will enable you to avoid loss of work from illness and keep you a productive member of society through many years.

Since population growth is dependent on a combination of birth rate and death rate, and if we are going to decrease the death rate, it seems only logical that we should also attempt to decrease the birth rate. In the recent past it was felt that all population problems could be solved by offering adequate birth control education or devices to the uneducated and underprivileged people of the world. This was naive, since it was based on the assumption that most pregnancies occurring among the underprivileged were unwanted. Numerous surveys have been made among people of different economic levels regarding what they feel to be the ideal family size. It is no great surprise to find that some people feel that three, four, or even five children would be an ideal and personally gratifying family size. Therefore, as one faces the reality of the situation, one must grant that sex education and family planning alone will not reduce our population growth. It will be necessary to offer motivation and encouragement to keep families small. Despite the previous statement, one must admit there are a large number of unwanted births in our population. These include not only the children of the young and unmarried, but also those married members of our population who, because of age or economics, desire no more children. From the data gathered by Larry Bumpass and Charles Westolf, and given in their essay in "The American Population Debate," one can assume that from one third to one fourth of the births in this country are unwanted. A chart of illegitimate births in 1967 is presented (see Appendix, Chart XXIX). Note the total illegitimate births of 318,100 and note that 46,400 were the fourth and fifth illegitimate children of a given female. If these children are wards of the state, does the state have some say as to the tolerable number?

I must confess that for the past 20 years I have had more than a passing interest in pediatrics. Children make up a fascinating segment of our population. Their response to their environment and to kindness or abuse offers a real promise that our people might be ideally molded under the proper circumstances. If a sick infant survives a serious illness, he represents a long-term survival and a truly significant contribution to society. Physicans are always proud to achieve a five-year survival from cancer in a patient at any age. Since cancer is primarily a disease of the aged, we may well be adding five years to a man who is already 70. This accomplishment is not to be frowned upon, but is slight when compared to the salvage of the life of an infant. There we can expect a survival of 70 years and a significant contribution to society.

It is because of our broad interest in medicine, and children in particular, that we offer the suggestion that some children would best not be born. This is especially true since there is a population problem. High-risk pregnancies, high-risk mothers, and high-risk situations that result in inadequate infants must first be identified; then all possible steps should be taken to avoid pregnancies in this group, which includes both married and unmarried females. Since our interest at this point is primarily in the child, the mother's status and her social problems are important. We must have healthy, low-risk newborns. What obviously is important is the mother's physical condition; she should be in first-class health. The father's health is relatively unimportant, providing he is genetically sound. Only paternal alcoholism and diabetes have been related to moderate increases in perinatal mortality. The mother, as we will point out time and again, is far more important in pregnancy than the father. The father is important only to start the process. After this, the mother provides not only half of the genetics, but a very important environment for the first nine months required to change the two initial cells into an infant.

If there is a case for compulsory birth control, as has been suggested by Dr. Edgar Chasteen in his essay in "The American Population Debate," I would suggest that physicians as well as demographers and politicians be consulted before any such compulsory program is initiated. Although freedom is very important to Americans, none of us is entirely free. It is well known that the right of free speech does not permit us to stand up in a crowded arena and shout "Fire!," and anyone who drives an automobile must follow the rules of the road for the good of the entire community. The same may well be true regarding the right to have children. If population needs to be controlled and if the birth rate needs to be reduced, obviously some segments of the population must be encouraged by education or by compulsion if necessary, to refrain from reproduction. In making such statements, one must be very careful not to select races or religions for genocide, but to select carriers of disease that affect infants. One such disease that carries a tremendously high infant mortality is diabetes. Diabetes crosses all race lines. It knows no religious barrier. Diabetic mothers are relatively small in number (2.3 per 1000 deliveries), but have a perinatal mortality of 18 per cent, which is approximately 6 times the accepted rate (Gordon).*

*H. H. Gordon. "The Infants of Diabetic Mothers," American Journal of Medical Science, 244: 129-144, July 1962.

Other authors, Benson and Babson in their book, "Management of High Risk Pregnancy and Intensive Care of the Neonate," hold that perinatal mortality may go up to 30 per cent! Diabetes that appears in females of childbearing age carries with it a high complication rate in pregnancy, and infants born to such parents also carry a high risk. At this point I would encourage all persons who have significant diabetes to refrain from having children. If they feel that they must raise children, these children should be adopted.

Polycystic kidney disease is another familial disease that greatly shortens the life of its victims. It is transmitted as a Mendelian genetic dominant characteristic. This disease is certainly serious enough to warrant stringent birth control measures by its victims. As in diabetes, it is frequently undiagnosed during the childbearing years.

Sickle cell disease is also a genetically transmitted disease that results in a great deal of morbidity and increased mortality to its victims. One black person in 12 carries the sickle cell trait. Therefore, the odds of two sickle cell trait carriers mating, necessary to produce a disease victim, are 1 in 144. This means that .7 per cent of all black families produce children with this disease. (Rare cases are found in whites.) It is estimated that in 1967 there were 1155 new cases. The victims of this disease have a median survival to age 20. In addition to this relatively short life expectancy, there is a great deal of crippling and many hospitalizations because of pain and disability. It is not uncommon for a young victim of sickle cell disease to have 40 to 50 hospital admissions during his relatively short life. Should a female sufferer of this disease reach the childbearing years and should she be unfortunate enough to become pregnant, the disease carries a maternal mortality of 10 to 14 per cent. The mortality rate of her infant is as high as 55 per cent. Because of the high maternal and infant risk with sickle cell disease Dr. Forte, writing in *The American Journal of Obstetrics and Gynecology* for October 1971, suggests that sterilization and/or abortion should be offered to all who suffer from this disability. Since this disease is virtually limited to the black race, to suggest genetic control may subject one to the criticism of advocating genocide. However, to date, this is the only means of controlling the disease; perhaps through medical research other means of control will be found. A geneticist, Dr. Neil Schemke, portrays this point with this illustration. Nearsightedness is a genetically transmitted error. In the days when men lived by hunting game, man's eyesight had to be good. The man born nearsighted might not survive—he starved or was cared for by his friends. His genetic problems were generally not carried forward to another generation. Today a pair of spectacles corrects this error completely and easily, enabling one to earn one's living normally. Now this genetic error is corrected so easily it is of no great importance. It would be wonderful if some simple correction could be found for sickle cell disease. Until such time we sincerely hope that young members of the black race will be checked for the sickle cell trail and seek genetic counseling before marriage.

In addition to the specific disease risks that have been mentioned above, it is well known that infant mortality and the obstetrical risk increases at both extremes of the child-bearing age. This specifically implies that teen-age pregnancy is a high-risk situation both for mother and baby. Dr. Hammouda in *The American Journal of Obstetrics and Gynecology* has reported a 10 per cent incidence of maternal toxemia in teen-age pregnancies. In addition, the premature infant birth rate is unacceptably high in the teen-age mother. In 1967 it was 17.2 per cent for mothers under 15 and 10.5 per cent for mothers in the 15-to-19 age group. Premature rates over 6 per cent are unacceptable. Likewise, the pregnancy of the female in her late 30's and early 40's carries a high statistical incidence of complication. Dr. Sydney Kane in *Obstetrics and Gynecology,* March, 1967, listed complications of pregnancy and compared the incidence for each age group. The complication rate was 34 per cent in older females, compared to 9 per cent for age 25. The incidence of chromosomal abnormalities such as Downs' syndrome (mongolism) and Turner's syndrome (ovarian absence) is known to increase with the age of the mother. Dr. Henry Nadler of Northwestern has reported that these abnormalities occur once in 2000 deliveries of mothers at age 25. At age 35 they occur once in 250 deliveries, at age 40 once in 120, and at age 45 once in each 45 deliveries. We are in a position to tell politicians and demographers that, if there is a necessity to lower the birth rate and if we want to keep infant mortality low and raise quality infants then pregnancy in the very young and in the older age groups should be very much discouraged. There is evidence that the live born infant mortality has improved in New York as a result of the high abortion rate in young females. If it is absolutely necessary to reduce the number of infants born, motherhood below the age of 20 and after 35 would be a prime candidate for prohibition. In 1967 women under age 20 delivered 605,038 babies, and women over 35 delivered 298,534.

The above statements are made with a high degree of medical honesty. We are being extremely naive if we feel that we can, by declaration, prevent females under the age of 20 and over the age of 35 from becoming pregnant. We can, and must, make readily available to these high-risk groups all possible birth control information. Ten years ago it would have been highly controversial to offer birth control advice to teen-age girls. There are some sections of the country and some religious groups even today who may construe such advice as a license for promiscuity. However, the unfortunate fact remains that many teen-age pregnancies occur and that these pregnancies occur even in the very early teen-age periods. No 13- or 14-year-old girl is physically or mentally prepared for motherhood. One of the greatest crimes that we as society in general or physicians in particular can perpetrate is to permit delivery to occur in this segment of our population. Even after having made the above statement, it is still naive to think that there is any way of preventing these age groups from becoming pregnant. This is true because a certain number of these females wish to become pregnant. It is even recognized among teen-agers that pregnancy may be desirable from their own standpoint; this is based on an ego need or may be a sign of rebellion or resentment against social and parental influence. There is no way a law could prevent this from occurring. If the law insisted that all such patients be aborted, they would still become pregnant and hide out until delivery time. It becomes apparent that, while compulsory birth control and compulsory abortion offer a fine solution in theory, there is no way such laws or rules can be enforced, or for that matter, even be made acceptable to our society.

Historically, Americans solve problems by one of two approaches. If the problem is a crisis—it sometimes seems that we survive from crisis to crisis—the usual tendency is to attempt to purchase a solution. We are frequently told that a crash program is needed for some worthy cause. Congress appropriates a large sum of money, and everyone expects the problem to be solved. This was how we built the atomic bomb. We needed to win the war, money was made available, and the bomb was developed. We have repeatedly tried to apply this line of reasoning to health and disease. Crash programs appear for cancer research and sums of money are requested for the mentally defective, all of which, it is assumed, will solve the problem. The population problem is so complex and so interwoven with religion, culture, and personal freedoms that no one seriously offers to place a price tag on its solution.

The second popular means of solving problems is through education. This country, from its inception, has fostered the belief that educating everyone not only makes life more acceptable for each individual person, but upgrades society as a whole. This ideal of our forefathers has done more for the development of the United States than any other concept. However, education takes time; if one is to change social or cultural patterns by education, one must think in terms of generations before these changes can become significant. Nevertheless, it seems proper that our people be given some insight into the problems of population. It is important that people realize that there are disadvantages to large populations and that these carry down to the individual. It should be pointed out that there are advantages to small families. The problem is not a simple one of numbers of people and food supply available. If these were the only factors involved, the problem would tend to be self-limiting. When a people outgrow the food supply, starvation and disease cut back on the population. This condition occurs in the underdeveloped nations, but only when outside influences are minimized. When outside influences reduce the death rate and incompletely restore the food supply, the problem becomes more malignant.

It has been pointed out that, while the United States represents only 6 per cent of the world's population, it consumes nearly 40 per cent of the world's resources. It has also been stated that if people all over the world were to adopt the standard of living we enjoy, the earth could support only a billion people instead of the nearly four billion that now exist. These figures imply that underdeveloped nations have population problems in terms of numbers of people and supplies of food, while the rich nations have a population problem in terms of overconsumption of the total resources available. Food is only one of these resources. In countries such as the United States and Canada, food production and population density present no great difficulty. Our problem is one of resources and consumption per person, not limited to food. Energy resources are more compelling than food at this time. From a resource-consumption standpoint, one American baby consumes an amount equivalent to 12.4 children in the rest of the world. W. H. Davis derived the term "Indian Equivalents" and offers a conservative estimate that one American baby uses 25 times as much of the earth's resources as an Indian infant. A rich country, therefore, has a population problem with far fewer people than the underdeveloped country. An energy crisis this decade may be a food crisis in the next decade. This is true because of our inflated standards of living. We would like to blame the oil companies or our government for our energy shortage but the real blame must rest with the large number of people each consuming excessively and demanding an endless supply of oil and its by-products.

As you read these pages, and if you read the books to which I have referred, particularly in regard to population problems, I am sure you will agree that we face a crisis. This is the first step in education. Once a problem is recognized, attempts at solution will be forthcoming. The mere recognition that something must be done does not in itself guarantee that constructive programs will be undertaken. Action is far more likely if the observed need is supported either by economic gain or legislative muscle. Thus, we now find ourselves in a position of recognizing a need and trying to develop the proper stimulus to see that this will be fulfilled. Certainly, the large family creates a financial problem to the parents as these children approach college age. There is no question that the father of such a family realizes that he has a tremendous financial handicap compared to the father of one, or possibly two, children. However, this realization, which is after the fact, does very little to eliminate the basic problem. The government might enter the picture by providing economic and legislative incentives for smaller families. One very simple method would be to eliminate the income tax deductions for more than two dependent children. Others have proposed that a couple should be granted a deduction for the first two children, but pay an additional tax for each additional child. This would serve as a financial incentive for small families. On first consideration, these methods seem quite logical. However, there are obvious drawbacks. First of all, the poor, who particularly need to be encouraged to reduce their numbers, would not be influenced by this technique, since they pay no tax. At the other extreme, the wealthy would not be deterred by this relatively small financial handicap, so their cooperation in the program could not be enlisted. Once again, it would be the middle-income group that would be forced to cooperate or suffer penalties for noncooperation. Another solution suggests that the government issue licenses for a certain number of children per couple; these would vary according to qualification. Health could be one of the qualifications, overall population numbers another. Ideal ratios, if such ratios exist, between different ethnic groups could even be arranged; in this way population could be controlled quite rigidly. The license system obviously has the problems of other forms of compulsory population control, but it is offered as a more extreme solution.

The strongest motivating force I can think of, other than the recognition that there is a population problem, stems from the fact that in the 1970's children are not the economic asset they were a century or even 50 years ago. They are now a distinct economic liability. Children bring happiness. They are lovable, and they support our egos. They assure the continuance of our species, but they are an economic liability. To rear a child from birth through college requires at least $25,000 (quoted figures may be as great as $75,000, depending upon the family's standard of living). In addition, as inflation increases, this cost may actually become greater than the increased income of the parents, particularly if the family is large. A 2 per cent increase in the cost of rearing a child would mean a 10 per cent increase if there were five children. The inflationary pressure alone would be difficult for the parents to tolerate.

Economic pressures have been felt by most families. Certainly, these pressures have been responsible, at least in part, for the downward trend in the birth rate that began in the late 1950's. This trend started before the "pill" was developed. So economics plays as big a role in the birth rate as any other single item. However, as I have repeatedly stated, the population problem is so complex that attention to only one aspect will not solve it. The poor especially may derive great personal satisfaction and personal identity from giving birth to children. Robert Cole's book *Children in Crises,* emphasizes this personal need in people of the inner city.

At the other end of the socioeconomic scale is a statement attributed to Golda Meir, the former Prime Minister of Israel. The general context of this statement was that she felt men were discriminated against in our society, and that discrimination against them was an act of God since they were not permitted to bear or rear children. An obstetrician friend of mine has been concerned with the overpopulation problem for a number of years and has done his bit to encourage women to have small families. He tells me that when a woman comes to him with that faraway look in her eye and states that she wishes to bear another child, it is virtually impossible to dissuade her. These statements demonstrate that an intangible aspect of the population problem relates to the female desire, not necessarily for sex, but for reproduction. Also, they make it perfectly evident that financial rewards or penalties cannot, in themselves, bring about a solution to the population problem.

It would be advantageous if we could find sources of gratification other than childbearing for the female members of society. Obviously, we would not want to be totally successful in this regard, or the race would become extinct. However, there seems to be little danger of this. Women's liberation may be making a very significant contribution to population control as a fringe benefit to the movement. If female members of our society are given equal opportunities in the professions, business, and in all other careers, there will be some women who find themselves so involved in these careers that childbearing will represent a significant handicap rather than emotional gratification. Therefore, as women become liberated from men economically, as birth control information and procedures become readily available, and as the economic pressure on the large family becomes more intense, it seems that the population problem will approach solution. Our falling birth rate seems to confirm this. If Dr. Ehrlich and others in this field continue to write and keep us aware of our problems, as I hope they will, it would seem that man may once more survive.

V. The First 28 Days

Infants and children exist in a world of life-threatening situations that are different from those of adults. Just as adults die from preventable diseases, so do children. The next four chapters of this book will be devoted to the age groups 0 through 14 years. I realize you may have limited interest in this young age group. If you have no interest in the younger years, please skip to Chapter IX. For those who have children or grandchildren, please continue with Chapter V.

If you move to Chapter IX and then finish the book, I hope you will be stimulated enough to return to the chapters involving infants and children. They are a fascinating segment of our population.

We gave the death rate of the first year of life at 2,233.1 per 100,000 births and commented that this was the highest rate until one reached the age of 65. Since approximately three-quarters of the deaths occurring in the first year occur in the first 28 days of life, it is obvious that this is indeed a very hazardous period. More precise figures are as follows: 79,028 deaths in the first year of life, with 58,127 occurring in the first 28 days. Since there are 1,851,323 deaths this same year, we are now looking at about 3 per cent of the deaths for 1967. Three per cent does not sound impressive, but when we can pinpoint these to just 28 days' time, we are referring to a very significant number.

Chart V is offered as a breakdown of the causes of death in the first 28 days of life.

Some explanation will be offered for each of the major categories. If you look at the massive data offered in *Vital Statistics of the United States* on infant mortality, you will not find these categories quite so well defined. I have also taken some license to combine categories. For instance, the record has a separate heading for hernia and intestinal obstruction. However, since I know by experience that virtually all hernias and intestinal obstructions in the first 28 days are caused by congenital anomalies, they are included in that group. I shall try to simplify and make the government's raw data more meaningful.

Congenital Anomalies

In this age of the medically sophisticated public, everyone knows something about birth defects. They represent errors in development of the fetus in the uterus. The embryonic development of an infant is very complicated; many processes occur simultaneously in this protected environment. Those of us who try to understand it are constantly amazed at how often everything turns out right when there are so many possibilities for error. The Master Planner of this project surely left very little for anyone to correct and much to amaze us. However, when there are so many combinations, once in a while one will come up wrong; the baby is less than perfect. Congenital heart lesions —blue babies and some that are not blue—clubfeet, spinal and spinal cord deformities, brain anomalies, severe metabolic defects, and many other disabilities fall into this wide heterogeneous group. Birth defects take lives at all ages. If you will refer back to Chart I (page 303), of the 15 leading causes of death you will find that birth defects occupy the 13th place. Approximately 18,000 people died of this problem, and most of these were under 5 years of age. Any salvage in this area, be it by prevention or cure, would result in many increased man years of productivity. This is a feature very difficult for statistics to reflect. On our charts and tables a death is a death, whether it occurs at age 1 or 100, yet it seems to me that to society there is a great difference. I will ask you repeatedly to take a hard look at these deaths in the childhood years.

The attitude of the medical profession as well as the public has changed markedly in the past century. Witchcraft is no longer of interest, but the fetal environment with its stresses of all types—psychological, chemical, physical, hormonal, or infectious—is one of the major medical fields of investigation in the 1970's. Attitudes on the part of all parties involved in pregnancy are very important. In this age of enlightenment, pregnancies should not be considered the curse of an evening of fun, but should be planned with the idea of placing this complex project of growth and development into the most favorable environment possible. Remember, this fetus must derive from his environment—his mother—all the chemicals, food materials, and oxygen necessary to convert from a single cell to a functioning human being of 15 trillion cells, all in a period of nine months. The fetus is not an isolated, insulated, incidental, coexisting object, but a developing human that must share the air the mother breathes and the food she eats if it is to survive. By the same token, this infant will share every drug the mother takes, whether it be for a headache or to indulge her desire for euphoria. This parasitic relationship is not all bad, for thus we can see that the fetus is well fed and that hormone and vitamin levels are maintained.

At this point we should review some of the agents associated with birth defects—teratogenic agents. Everyone remembers thalidomide, which appeared in the early 60's. This drug was basically a sedative and was apparently a good product—for its purpose. However, it was given to a certain number of pregnant women, probably for morning sickness, with disastrous results. Phocomelia, children without extremities or with only flippers where extremities should be, resulted. However, even in the years when thalidomide was at peak usage it accounted for only about 1 per cent of the deformed infants born at that time; nevertheless, it so incensed physicians and the public that great effort has been spent since that time to protect the fetus against drugs of all types. This one disaster did more to awaken everyone to the real relationship between the fetus, the mother, and the outside world than any other event in the last 50 years.

We divide teratogenic agents into three types; chemical, physical, or infectious. Needless to say, each of these categories occupies a rather large area. As you are all aware, virtually every drug that is now placed on the market is checked to be certain it is not teratogenic. The chemical agents now produce relatively few numbers of congenital defects. Unfortunately, there are so many new chemical agents with which all people come into contact that it is difficult to analyze which may be of significant harm to the infant. Despite the great inconvenience to the drug manufacturers and to the physicians, this type of research or detective work into the effects of all drugs must continue. Our society cannot afford or tolerate another thalidomide incident.

Another group of chemicals to which all people are exposed comprises those that are not intended for human consumption. Because of this, they have not been as carefully checked by the Federal Drug Administration as those intended for human consumption. These drugs include pesticides, fertilizers, and chemical purifiers. In the last few years we have heard ecological arguments against the use of DDT, the chlorinated hydrocarbon compounds, and even nitrate and nitrite fertilizers. These chemicals have been very important in increasing land productivity and control of predatory insects. Once they are placed in our environment, they invariably find their way to man. Whether these chemicals in small amounts may produce birth defects is unknown. Certainly, their presence in the mother can do no conceivable good to the developing fetus, yet the incidence of birth defects has not appreciably increased since these compounds have been introduced into our environment. Regulation of these chemicals is under way; it is therefore hoped that their amount in the environment will not increase. Continued vigilance in this area must be maintained by physicians, ecologists, and government agencies.

Of the physical agents with which humans may come in contact during pregnancy that are known to be teratogenic, the outstanding example is radiation. The best general rule is that no one who is pregnant should be subjected to any form of high-energy radiation, more specifically, the X ray. Nevertheless, we are all aware of exceptions that warrant the risk of this exposure. The classic example of this risk is pelvimetry, for there are times when the obstetrician questions whether the maternal pelvis is adequate to permit birth of the fetus. In such a case, as labor starts, one of the most accurate ways of measuring a pelvis is by X ray. Measurement of the pelvis by X ray can be done quite safely as delivery time approaches. We know that the teratogenic effect of all the agents we have listed previously depends on exposure in the first trimester—the first 3 months of pregnancy. By the time the mother goes into labor, the fetus is already formed and no teratogenic effects can be imposed thereon. We prefer to keep all exposure to a minimum; during pelvimetry, as small an area of the fetal body as possible is exposed. Thus, every attempt is made to keep the fetal dose small, even after a teratogenic effect is no longer probable. There are also times when ultrasound techniques can be used instead of X ray. At this time we feel ultrasound is safer than the X ray; as it improves and becomes more available, it may replace the X ray for obstetrical patients. Ultrasound may be used to plot intrauterine growth.

There are times when patients are exposed to X ray before knowing that they are pregnant. When such exposure occurs to the very early fetus, there is always great soul-searching on the part of the physician and patient when the true situation becomes known. It is not uncommon for us to be questioned as to whether abortion may be indicated in such an instance.

To evaluate exposure and settle the question of abortion, one must know when the study was done, the amount of exposure that occurred, and what areas of the mother were exposed. It is also important to take into account the desires of the patient. There is no arbitrary number of rads (the unit for the absorbed dose of radiation) to which the mother is exposed that will result with any degree of certainty in a deformed fetus. We know that the incidence of some types of congenital deformity in babies is approximately 2 to 4 per cent of all pregnancies without the addition of any known teratogen. From experimental animals we know that, in order to double the birth defect rate, we need to expose the subjects to somewhere in the range of 50 rads. There are no diagnostic procedures that result in this strength of exposure to the maternal pelvis. However, there is no substitute for honest discussion between physician and patient at this point. Certainly, if the patient has received more than 10 rads, in this day of legal and liberal abortion a termination of pregnancy may be considered. I have not yet recommended abortion in any instance for radiation exposure; also, I have yet to witness the birth of an infant with such a congenital defect. The Europeans have been more liberal in their indications for abortion in regard to radiation exposure than the Americans. The 10-rad figure is one that they have used.

We have learned more about radiation as a teratogenic agent and its general biological effect as a result of the atomic explosions at Hiroshima and Nagasaki. The American and Japanese governments have spent a great deal of time and money in attempts to follow all patients who were exposed to radiation from those bombs. A certain number of pregnant females in various stages of gestation were, of course, exposed to one massive dose of radiation. The stillborn rate was considerably higher than normal after that exposure, and the rate rose as the exposure increased. The same was true of the incidence of congenital anomalies, although the increase in this area was not as great as the increase in still births, indicating that radiation did kill the fetus, and the fetus was aborted in a number of instances. The only consistent birth defect reported was reduced skull size; these babies apparently received over 200 rads—at least 100 times the usual diagnostic X ray dosage. There have also been reports of increased incidence of childhood leukemia in infants exposed to radiation before birth. There are conflicting studies in this regard. Dr. R. Gibson, from Roswell Park Institute, Buffalo, feels that childhood leukemia is related to multiple-risk factors, of which one is radiation to the mother before or during pregnancy.

The third of our major teratogens is infectious disease. No one knows how many infectious agents are important in the formation of abnormal babies. Research is being carried on in an attempt to identify organisms that can traverse the placenta and either directly produce illness in the fetus or give rise to antibodies that can traverse the placenta and secondarily involve the fetus. Probably the best known infectious teratogen is rubella (measles). Syphilis has been known for many generations to produce blindness and mental defectives and actively to infect the unborn baby. Cytomegalic inclusion disease is a viral illness known to produce central nervous system damage to the baby. While it may on occasion produce death or severe abnormalities, its role in producing less serious defects is now under active investigation. Toxoplasmosis is also known to produce brain damage in infants. This is apparently not a virus, but a sporazoan parasite.

Of the mentioned infectious agents that produce known

fetal abnormalities, rubella and syphilis are the most common; fortunately, both of these can be prevented. Rubella vaccine is available and quite effective. Because of this, we can hope that the rubella syndrome of the newborn baby will soon be a thing of the past. Rubella vaccine, while effective in preventing rubella, is also a teratogenic agent. It should not be given to pregnant women or to women at any time less than 120 days prior to conception. Rubella, like radiation, is most dangerous in the first trimester of pregnancy. When active rubella can be proven in this gestation period, the incidence of birth defects goes up to as high as 75 per cent. For this reason, rubella or rubella vaccine in early pregnancy has become a medical indication for abortion. Babies born of a mother infected with rubella may have a number of anomalies, the most common of which are cataracts, resulting in blindness; deafness; and congenital heart disease. It also seems that these children thrive very poorly and that their disability extends beyond the specific anomalies mentioned above. Studies have shown that these babies have fewer cells per organ than normal. This is only one of the areas where good maternal prenatal care can be very influential in preventing birth defects.

There is no vaccination for syphilis. It is a disease that has been with us for centuries and probably will remain for many centuries to come. It is a treatable disease; any female who is pregnant and who has or has had the disease requires reevaluation during the course of her pregnancy. Here again the role of the physician in the prenatal care of the patient becomes important. This disease is in general easily recognized, and because of the efficient treatment available congenital syphilis is, for the most part, vanishing from our newborn nurseries. Unfortunately, it has not completely disappeared; just when we feel confident that this problem is approaching control, there seems to be a renewed outbreak. Vigilance on the part of the attending physician is probably the most important preventive measure of this illness. Some obstetricians insist on testing for syphilis on the patient's first visit and again as delivery time approaches. It is quite possible for a patient to be free of the disease early in pregnancy, but to contract the disease before delivery time and thereby infect the baby late in the course of his development. It seems that infections acquired late in pregnancy are somewhat less disastrous than those acquired earlier.

The other two infectious agents we have listed, toxoplasmosis and cytomegalic inclusion disease, have considerable similarity. Both are known to be the cause of intrauterine infection. Both have been known to produce severe damage to the infant, primarily to the central nervous system. Both are known to be implicated in repeated or habitual abortion. Despite the fact that these organisms have been implicated in severe brain damage in infants, the number of children severely affected is relatively small. This is true despite the fact that these organisms are relatively common in nature. We know that the cytomegalic inclusion virus is frequently found in the birth canal and saliva. It therefore seems unusual that it should produce such severe anomalies on some occasions and have no effect on others. We are beginning to recognize less severe forms of this disease such as deafness and mild mental retardation. At this time I would not even try to guess the importance of this virus ten years in the future.

Toxoplasmosis also occurs quite frequently in nature. It has been stated that as high as 30 per cent of the population may have antibodies against this organism. The presence of antibodies seems to be geographically dependent. There are areas in the Southwest where antibodies in people are quite unusual, and there are other parts of the world where they are very common. Toxoplasma gondii is an intracellular parasitic-type organism. It can cause severe damage to infants or to older children. As with cytomegalic inclusion disease, there has been a great deal of research attempting to correlate it with other birth defects, particularly mental retardation. It must be admitted that there is some statistical evidence to associate both of these organisms with mental retardation, but the evidence is not overwhelming. However, the implications persist, and for this reason both cytomegalic inclusion disease and toxoplasma are considered very significant organisms worthy of further investigation.

Suggestions as to prevention of infection with these organisms are limited. There have been some rather interesting observations made in regard to toxoplasma. This organism may be transmitted to humans by cats, which are known to be frequent carriers of the organism. Perhaps some scientific evidence will confirm the old wives' tale that expectant mothers should not be around cats. At any rate, our only suggestion to avoid these infections is to avoid patients who are known to have been involved with these diseases and possibly to avoid pets, particularly cats. The advice of the attending obstetrician in these areas should be followed. With more study, the patterns of these diseases, their treatment, and possibly immunizations can be developed.

Since we know that viruses and various organisms can produce disastrous effects on the unborn fetus, all of us have the recurring thought that more benign infections that strike us all with little or no morbidity may be important in the early months of gestation. Probably all maternal illnesses have some effect on the developing fetus. The severity of this effect depends on the severity of the disease, the resistance of the mother, and the stage of fetal development at which the infection occurs. Polio has been associated with fetal neuromuscular abnormalities. Mumps has been associated with heart muscle abnormalities. The herpes, or fever blister, virus may result in small, immature babies.

Asian flu early in pregnancy has been associated with skull and spinal canal anomalies.

No one can accurately estimate the percentage of fetal abnormalities and deaths that may be related to these chemical, physical, and infectious agents. At this time 25 per cent would be a generous estimate. This means that most birth defects are primarily genetic in origin, but with some other physical, chemical, or infectious contributory factor. Those wishing a more complete list will find it in Chart XXX in the Appendix.

We have said nothing as yet about fetal monitoring or surveillance. It is part of prenatal care. Indeed, in a broad sense, all of prenatal care is fetal and maternal surveillance. I shall use the term "fetal surveillance" to describe some very exciting investigations now going on in the field of prenatal care. Attempts are being made to study the chromosome structure and the biochemical composition of the cells of the unborn baby. In this way it should be possible to identify many abnormalities prior to birth. A few drops of the amniotic fluid in which the fetus floats are removed by a needle inserted through the mother's abdomen and into the uterine cavity. The risk of this maneuver has been shown to be quite small. The cells in this fluid are fetal cells. The fluid can be studied for its chemical characteristics and the cells studied directly, or they can be cultured for additional chromosome studies.

Chromosome studies are laborious, and some of the biochemical studies are complex, but the potential reward is promising. The list of fetal disorders that can be diagnosed in this manner is steadily expanding. As long ago as October 1970, Dr. Kurt Hirschhorn reported at a symposium on birth defects and the environment that some 27 different fetal disorders could be diagnosed in this manner.

While it does not seem feasible to carry out these detailed

studies on all pregnancies, we know some high-risk pregnancies will occur. These can be monitored. The identification of severe defects prior to birth may significantly alter the management of that pregnancy. This is one more example of where the option of quality in life can be offered.

Certain Diseases of the Newborn

The statistical entry that covers the largest number of deaths in the first 28 days has a vague title. It is particularly vague to people not associated with the care of infants. This category is made up of the entities included in Chart VI.

CHART VI

Certain Diseases of Newborn

Birth injuries
Postnatal asphixia & atelectasis
Pneumonia of newborn
Diarrhea of newborn
Other infections of newborn

(Neonatal disorders arising from maternal disorders)
Hemolytic disease of newborn
Hemorrhagic disease of newborn
Nutrition maladjustments of newborn
Unqualified immaturity

Prematurity and its complications, especially respiratory distress syndrome, are the leading cause of death during the first 28 days of life. Reducing the number of deaths in this category offers a challenge to physicians and hope to the public. There is no question that this can be significantly decreased. This rate of 24 per 100,000 was reduced to 19 per 100,000 in 1971, and in 1972 the decline continued. This improvement in mortality figures is, to a large extent, attributable to a group of physicians who specialize in the care of newborn infants, neonatalogists. Intensive-care nurseries have been developed in virtually every major city; such an intensive-care nursery may be warranted in hospitals where over 3000 deliveries occur per year. In hospitals with less than 3000 deliveries per year, infants are frequently transferred to a highly specialized nursery that can be shared with other institutions. Under these conditions, the premature infant is receiving medical care superior to that available in the past.

Unfortunately, no matter how good a job the physician does in caring for this premature infant, that infant will not be as fine a specimen as he might have been had he been a full-term delivery. Once again I am pointing to the fact that we, as physicians, are treating results and not preventing the real cause of the difficulty. Some energies have been directed to the prevention of prematurity, but they are not nearly as aggressive as our attempts to care for and treat the permature infant.

Even with our improved mortality figures, there is some question whether we are doing society a real favor with intensive care of the premature infant. Some leaders in this field have suggested that we are salvaging infants that may have had severe brain damage because of their disease and making of these infants, by means of good care, normal children. This is certainly to the credit of society. On the other hand, prematures that ordinarily would have died are being salvaged, but if this salvage is less than complete, there may be significant physical and mental inadequacies in this salvaged infant. The question may justly be raised: Is it better to have a live infant that will be mentally or physically handicapped or should we willingly have accepted the death of the very small premature as a charitable act of God? No one at this point can honestly answer that question. Dr. L. O. Lubchenco, reporting in *The Journal of*

Pediatrics for March 1972, has a 10-year follow-up on babies 3.5 pounds or less. The shocking truth is that only 30 per cent were normal, 66 per cent were handicapped (50 per cent severely), and 43 per cent were mentally retarded. Most of us hope that this gloomy report is not applicable to the entire nation. I am told that the group at Toronto Babies Hospital will soon be in print with better statistics. The Stanford group is also more optimistic.

A report out of the University of Chicago gives results similar to the Denver data. Denver is at an atmospheric disadvantage compared to most other cities. We can assume that over the next five years there will be statistics available to tell us more about the children being salvaged in this group.

The obvious and overwhelming statistic is that nearly 80 per cent of the children who die in this category do so because they were born prematurely. To anyone interested in preventive medicine, herein lies the hope of salvage of at least 30,000 infants per year. Premature births must be prevented if we are to realize significant gains in this area.

Understandably, the terms prematurity and low birth weight have been used interchangeably. However, to use them thus is hardly defensible. Premature babies usually are low in birth weight, but low-birth-weight babies are not necessarily premature. To clarify this point, human gestation requires 280 days. A baby born at the 200th day will certainly be premature and will be of low birth weight. However, should the baby be born at 310 days, he will be post-term in gestational age, but may actually be of low birth weight if his intrauterine growth and development have been slower than normal. A child born at 280 days, which would be the normal time of delivery, may weigh only three to four pounds and show clinical signs of malnutrition. This, then, would be a low-birth-weight, full-term infant. Since the date of conception is rarely known with accuracy, we have in the past used the weight of a baby as the index of its maturity. Virtually all of the medical and statistical literature classes any infant under 2500 grams—5 pounds, 8 ounces—as premature. Therefore, when discussing prematurity, this division is made on the basis of the indicated weight. Physicians who are expert in this field agree that the weight division for premature infants is an artificial one. The fetal length, measured from the crown of the head to the heel, and circumference of the head are probably more accurate ways of measuring gestational age than is the weight of the infant. However, at this point virtually all statistics are based on the weight division of infants. Therefore, those of us who are interested students in the field must also use the 2500-gram division, but admit that there are more ideal ways of differentiating the premature from the term infant.

Prevention of Prematurity

It is difficult to give an ideal birth weight for an infant. A study of death statistics implies that the infant most likely to survive the rigors of the first 28 days is a child with a calculated gestational age of 280 days, a birth weight of between six and one-half and eight pounds, and a heel-to-crown length of 20 inches. Certainly, many infants who survive very well are smaller or larger, but this is the age and size of the infant with the best chance for survival. A prolonged gestational period and a post-mature baby is a not infrequent occurrence, and it is associated with increased mortality. Since it is less common than prematurity and we are trying to find preventable causes of infant death, evaluation of the premature offers far more opportunities for salvage than does consideration of the post-mature infant. Since there is no single cause of prematurity, there can obviously be no single preventive measure to avoid premature delivery.

It has been stated that prematurity can be reduced with good prenatal care. This is true—to a point. Certainly, one of the causes of prematurity is illness of the mother. If the mother can be kept free of disease and all complications during her pregnancy, the infant has the best opportunity to be born at term. In this sense, the physician caring for the mother during her pregnancy can be very helpful in preventing premature labor. Diet during pregnancy is also important. The mother must not be permitted to gain a large amount of weight. She must nevertheless eat adequately so that the fetus is supplied with all its nutritional needs during this developing period.

Probably even more important than prenatal care is the health of the mother even before she conceives. In this sense we are using health as it relates to ideal reproductive function. The potential young mother's health should be evaluated with regard to all of the factors related to the nutrition of the unborn infant.

Good medical prenatal care is available to everyone in this country. It is available either through the private practice sector of our economy or through our university and general hospital clinics. There is no doubt that the professional skills available to the poor through these two types of organizations are excellent. I am also convinced that most men in private practice do a good job caring for the pregnant female.

Despite the fact that medical prenatal care of good quality is available at all levels of society, there is no question about the increased frequency of low-birth-weight infants in the lower socioeconomic groups. This fact has been emphasized by many authors and can be determined from the vital statistic figures. Rather than recite general statistics in this area, let me relate a personal experience. During the last year I have had the opportunity to do the diagnostic radiology for two separate institutions. The first hospital, in which I have been working for four years, is a general private hospital of approximately 600 beds. The patients are generally middle-class suburban people who have an average to better-than-average income. There are approximately 2400 deliveries each year in this hospital. The rate of low-birth-weight infants in this environment is 5.8 per cent, and in this group of low-birth-weight infants we have had severe respiratory distress in 2.19 per 1000 births.

The second institution is a children's hospital. No deliveries occur here; however, its intensive-care ward receives desperately ill children from the entire metropolitan area. However, the main source of its referrals is the municipal hospital, which is next door. It was painfully apparent that we were seeing many more sick premature infants than I had anticipated, and certainly far more than we were seeing at my primary hospital. Therefore, statistically speaking, we eliminated the referrals from outlying small community hospitals, but kept statistics from the municipal hospital next door. They deliver approximately 2300 babies per year; the low-birth-weight rate is 12.5 per cent, with an incidence of severe respiratory distress in 15.9 babies per 1000. In short, the low-birth-weight rate in the municipal hospital was slightly more than twice that of the suburban community hospital, and severe respiratory distress was eightfold greater in the lower socioeconomic group.

There can be no denying the fact that some significant difference in the socioeconomic patterns of the two groups must account for this difference in low-birth-weight infants and even more importantly in the illness to which they are predisposed by the low birth weight. Prenatal medical care, although available to those in lower socioeconomic groups, was not always used. It was not uncommon for a patient to deliver on the first visit to the municipal hospital. This did not occur at the private hospital. Both hospitals had patients with variations in age, although young deliveries were more numerous at the municipal hospital than at the private institution.

Despite such attempts to explain the differences, we are seemingly forced to accept the idea that preconception health is vital to all would-be mothers and that in the lower socioeconomic groups, while prenatal medical care may be available, preconception health is not up to par. Scientific proof of this is hard to adduce, but practicing obstetricians accept it as common knowledge. This may be related to diet, infection, sanitation, stress, or combinations of any of these factors. It seems that the health of the female from her own birth to the time she conceives is even more important than prenatal care. We need to instill in every female inclined to have children the idea that her health must be as ideal as possible prior to conception. In this way she can provide the ideal environment for the fetus and, we hope, carry it to full term.

Preconception Health

In our discussion of peconception health, we have opened a Pandora's box, for we are not only talking of good general health, but are speaking in terms of health directed toward a given goal: the delivery of a full-term, normal infant.

Some of the steps necessary to achieve this goal should be apparent from our previous discussion. Virtually all young women think of their role as mothers early in life. Prior to conception and hopefully even before marriage the female should find a physician and discuss her health as it pertains to the important role of childbearing.

Freedom From Disease. There is no question that the most important determination in evaluating health is ruling out the presence of disease. Finding this abnormality is a function of the physician. He will take your history, do a physical examination, and perform the laboratory and X ray tests that he feels are indicated. While the absence of disease and good health are not entirely synonymous, certainly we cannot have good health in the presence of disease. There is a special reason why freedom from disease is important in the preconception period. We are trying to establish an ideal environment for the fetus. It is vital for your physician to know about syphilis, tuberculosis, heart disease, and diabetes at this time. If any of these diseases are found, their severity must be established and advice and treatment offered for your specific condition. I plead with diabetics to seek genetic counseling and seriously consider adoption rather than pregnancy if a family life is to be planned.

Freedom From Transmittable Diseases. This may sound like a repetition of the previous paragraph, but there is a distinct difference. A female desiring to have children may be in good health by all of our criteria and still carry genes that result in transmission of a disease to the offspring. A classic example of this is hemophilia; only males actually have the disease, which is genetically transmittted through maternal lines. We have previously mentioned sickle cell disease, polycystic disease, and diabetes. There are many others less common—osteogenesis imperfecta (fragile bones), some types of mental retardation, and growth abnormalities. A high incidence of birth defects of any type in either side of the family should be enough to encourage you and your physician to seek genetic counseling prior to conception. Such counseling does not assure you of a normal baby, but lets you enter the pregnancy aware of the statistical possibility of having a normal or abnormal infant. There will be times when the family histories are such that the parents will be advised not to have children. My plea to you is to heed such advice when it is given.

Freedom From Undue Mental Or Physical Stress. This is a vague category, very difficult for your physician to evaluate. It is probably best evaluated by you, providing you will do some honest soul-searching. We have come a long way since the days of witchcraft. We do not seriously feel that mothers "mark" their infants. However, the high-risk pregnancies occur under many emotional situations. It is well known that illegitimacy increases the risk of pregnancy. It is also recognized that insecurity may increase the risk. This insecurity may be in the forms of threatened divorce, financial disaster, or physical threat to the mother. If such insecurity and instability exist in the home, it does not create the ideal environment in which the fetus may grow and develop or in which the child may properly be reared.

The Question Of Diet. In the course of preconception evaluation the dietary history and habits of the would-be mother should be evaluated. This may be done by the physician or by the patient herself, provided she will look at her diet objectively. The dietary requirements will be somewhat different for each individual. Obesity is inconsistent with good health at any age. If an obese female wishes to become pregnant, a vigorous period of sensible weight control should be instituted and the pregnancy delayed until this disease process, obesity, is under control. The American diet is a notoriously poor one, since it is high in fats and sugars and tends to be low in proteins and vitamins. Since diet is such an integral part of health, a few comments are pertinent. Dr. E. Perry Crump of the Pediatric Department of Meharry Medical College lists a "significant degree of malnutrition" as one of the causes of low-birth-weight infants among ghetto dwellers. This is not acute malnutrition, but chronic malnutrition incident to a marginal existence. Malnutrition is not always economic in its origin, but may reflect poor habits or poor judgment on the part of the young female adult. In many instances malnutrition is a difficult entity to define. I am convinced that we do not understand all of the possible causes for malnutrition. The body is such a complex chemical machine that it undoubtedly has many components and combinations of components with which we are not totally familiar. We know that the body needs vitamins, minerals, and proteins, but perhaps we do not comprehend the proportions of each that are ideal or understand the storehouse that may be called upon to supply these vital elements when short-term or medium-term shortages exist. Part of our program of preconception health should be not only to maintain an adequate diet, but to be sure that any reserve storehouses are adequately filled.

Some women can and should lose weight consistently during pregnancy and can do this with complete safety to the baby. Other females should gain more than the 20 to 25 pounds that have constituted our previous goal in an attempt to prevent the low-birth-weight infant. Dr. Tom Brewer has reported some very exciting data. The average birth weight of black babies in his practice is 7.4 pounds, compared to the national average of 5.9 pounds. This has been brought about by careful nutrition of the mother during pregnancy. He avoids the use of drugs and dangerous restrictive diets and has founded an organization called Society for Protection of the Unborn through Nutrition (SPUN). His organization is in a position to be a real leader in the elimination of low-birth-weight infants.

Another bit of data that seems important has been reported from Canada. Simply adding 30 gm (1 ounce) of protein per day to the diet of pregnant females reduces the premature rate by 50 per cent and the mortality by more than one third. This again emphasizes the value of adequate nutrition in the nine months of pregnancy. No one has tried adding 30 gm of protein per day to the diet of females one year prior to pregnancy as well as during the period of pregnancy. By my line of reasoning this would reduce the mortality even more.

Well-trained nutritionists should be available in every medical community. However, you should be warned that some nutritionists have become "food fadists." Some available books are of questionable value and others actually may be harmful. Dr. Jean Meyer, a nutritionist who writes a syndicated column in many newspapers, is truly excellent. His advice is sound.

Should exercise and physical conditioning be part of a preconception program? This is an area of advice that is relatively new to would-be mothers. There are limited scientific data to buttress the concept, but all we know of health and fetal environment would logically support it. It is all a part of our concept of good preconception health. Since the fetus is utterly dependent upon the function of the maternal heart and lungs, it seems logical that we should do everything possible to have the heart and lungs both free of disease and functioning efficiently. In order to achieve this, a physical fitness program should be undertaken. In this regard the work done by Dr. Kenneth Cooper must be considered as the best available. He is one of the few physicians who have seriously undertaken the evaluation and measurement of health. There are many experts in the field of physical fitness and health. The Europeans, especially the Scandinavians, have been active in this field for years. In this country names like Samuel Fox III, Thomas Cureton, William Haskell, John Boyer, H. K. Hellerstein, Albert Kattus, Jr., Robert Bruce, Ernst Simonson, L. E. Morehouse, Ernst Jokl and many others have done good work in this field. Kenneth Cooper, however, took his case to the public and wrote an understandable book that has weaned thousands of people away from the sedentary life. His book, *Aerobics*, is good. His second book, *The New Aerobics,* offers information in regard to female fitness. Most of Dr. Cooper's work was done with U. S. military personnel; only in his second volume does he give us some criteria by which to measure the physical fitness of women. For a female under the age of 30 to be classed as being in "good physical condition" she must be able to travel a distance of 1.35 miles or more in 12 minutes. This may be a relatively difficult hurdle. A third book, *Aerobics For Women* by Dr. Cooper and his wife, makes no change in criteria for physical fitness from his previous standards. If such standards can be attained, there would seem to be little question that the blood supply to the developing fetus should be adequate. During the time we are establishing the ideal environment for the future fetus, we expect the would-be mother to walk and jog 20 to 30 minutes per day. Problems that arise in some pregnancies will require restriction of this type of activity. I am referring especially to the female who habitually aborts early in pregnancy. It has been felt for years that these patients should be kept at rest during early pregnancy. I cannot help but feel that, if the female is in good physical condition prior to conception, these spontaneous abortions and miscarriages may be less of a problem. Start your program before pregnancy!

We intend to say very little about drug habits as we commonly understand them, for we assume that anyone seriously interested in giving birth to a first-class infant will not be involved in such foolhardy practice. However, some information in regard to the effects of drug addiction on pregnancy may be of interest. One of the best articles on this subject appeared in *Pediatrics* for August 1971, written by Carl Zelson, M.D. and several colleagues at New York Medical College. They quoted their experience in the Metropolitan Hospital in New York over the ten-year period from 1960 through 1969. During this time 384 infants were born to 382 addicts. Forty-nine per cent of this group of babies weighed less than 2500 grams. This represents a sevenfold increase in the incidence of low-birth-weight infants. Of these infants 67.4 per cent had withdrawal symptoms; of those who had withdrawal symptoms, 68 per cent required active medical treatment. The instance of congenital defects was not above normal. The fetal death rate was 3.6 per cent, which is approximately twice the usual infant death rate. Of interest was the fact that no respiratory distress syndrome occurred in this group of babies. This is important medical information. It may be that drug addicts will teach us something of value about newborns. By all standards of logic and reasoning, no potential mother can contribute anything to the total well-being of her infant if she has such habits.

Fads may involve anything. Dietary fads have been notorious for generations. Bizarre diets may be used to lose weight, improve complexion, or achieve other ends. Fads of this type have no place in maternal health or fetal well-being. It does not take much imagination to realize that food fads may be very dangerous; others may be unnecessary. It has been suggested that the next consumer fraud may be that of "organically grown food." There is certainly no way, by the time the food reaches the market, that anyone can determine whether it was grown in an organically pure environment or in a standard manner. We may seriously question whether it makes any difference. The only problem that may arise is that of pesticides, and the government seems to be aggressively studying this area. Any change in our incidence of congenital anomalies or fetal distress will be pursued with vigor from all approaches.

Other more common habits that are recognized as deleterious to health need to be discussed with particular reference to pregnancy. It has been estimated that 25 per cent of women in the childbearing age groups smoke cigarettes. It was reported in medical literature as early as 1957 that low-birth-weight infants were born twice as frequently by smoking mothers as by nonsmokers. In 1964 the Surgeon

General reported to the nation that smoking was especially dangerous during pregnancy. Women who smoke 30 or more cigarettes per day have infants that weigh at least half a pound less than those of their nonsmoking sisters. In a relatively extensive study done in 1967, the number of infants born at the 36-week gestation time or earlier was found to be 7.5 per cent in smoking mothers and only 5.8 per cent in nonsmoking mothers. Since the fetus is wholly dependent upon the mother for its oxygen supply, any interference with oxygen exchange at the maternal level logically should be avoided. As indicated in the data above, smoking harms the fetus and creates additional risks for the infant. Other considerations with respect to oxygen supply may also be logically commented upon at this time. It is well known that the oxygen tension at high altitudes is less than at sea level. It is also known that people who live at high altitudes compensate for this by having a larger number of red blood cells available to carry the available oxygen. It seems logical that, if a female moves from sea level to the mountainous areas, a significant period of adaptation should be allowed before she enters into a pregnancy.

Another habit that deserves comment here is that of consuming alcohol. Data of the type reported with tobacco usage are, to my knowledge, not available with respect to alcohol consumption. We can only state what is known with respect to the physiology of alcohol consumption and assume that there will be the same effects on the developing fetus. Even drinking in the amounts usually classified as "social drinking" have been reported to produce brain cell death in the consumer—in this case the mother. Whether death thus occurs because of a direct neurotoxic effect or because of some interference with oxygen transfer is not known. In any event, it would seem poor judgment for the would-be mother to risk this self-indulgence when her baby is rapidly developing its brain. We do not know that the infant brain, as it develops, is more sensitive to reduced oxygen tension or to drugs than is the adult brain, but logic implies that this is true. However, it would be extremely difficult scientifically to determine whether infants born of mothers who were occasional drinkers had fewer brain cells than those born of mothers who were nondrinkers. Since science finds it difficult to answer this question categorically, we should accept the fact that alcohol can do the fetus no benefit and may produce damage to the growing infant. Our advice, therefore, to the would-be mother seems rather evident. Like tobacco, alcohol should be avoided completely during pregnancy. Since we are also talking of preconception health, it seems proper to state that both should be avoided during this period, as well. As our discussion of health and disease and its effect upon mortality rates continues, we shall be forced to the conclusion that alcohol and tobacco should be avoided in the interest of good health at all times.

Maligancy

Thirty-seven deaths were listed as attributable to malignancy in the first 28 days of life. Malignancy occurs and kills throughout the entire life span of the human, just as birth defects can take lives at all ages, from the newborn to the octogenarian. I was surprised to see that as many as 37 children died of malignancy in the first 28 days. I see no possible way of reducing the figure. These are children who are born with tumors and are incurable at birth. It may be that, as we learn more about the natural history of neoplastic disease, we will be able to predict that certain mothers give rise to infants contaminated with this disease. If that day comes, preventive measures may be developed. At the moment, we can only be thankful that no more than 37 children suffered death from this cause. Malignancy will become a major portion of our discussion as our study of death reaches the middle and later years. Infections, accidents, and homicides will aso be discussed later.

VI. The Period of Continuing Danger From 1 Month to 1 Year

The high risk of the first 28 days has now been well documented, but all risk does not, of course, end after the first month. However, there is a striking drop in the number of deaths that occur as the infant grows older. Chart VII demonstrates this drop. Note that the number of deaths during the second month of life is nearly ten times the number that occur during the eleventh month.

In our reference on infant mortality each death occurring in each of these months is attributed to one of 55 causes. This is excellent for the physician or interested researcher, but too detailed for others. We will group many of these causes together as we did for the first 28 days. It also is impracticable for us to consider each month separately. We offer Chart VIII for the causes of death for the infant from age 28 days to one year without regard to month.

After our previous discussions of population problems, preconception health, and the first 28 days of life, Chart VIII appears straightforward. We have already discussed birth defects and what hope there is for preventing them. These same disorders carry forward into the first year of life and continue to produce fatalities. Most of the birth defect fatalities in this period of life are attributed to heart disease or defects of the spine and central nervous system. A great deal is being done medically to correct these lesions. With good medical care we can hope to reduce the death rate from birth defects, but prevention of the defects themselves has rather limited potential at the moment. Genetic counseling is emphasized for families that have a high incidence of birth defects. Remember that 75 per cent of birth defects are genetic in type and that the other 25 per cent are caused by invaders of the fetal environment.

"Certain diseases of the newborn" were listed in the previous chapter. Prematurity claimed an additional 889 infants between the 28th day and the end of the first year. This gives us a staggering death toll for this entry in our chart of 48,271. As a matter of interest, 22 more patients died in this category between the ages of 1 and 5. Because of the small number of people dying of this entity beyond the first year, it will no longer appear as an entry in any of our statistical charts.

Infections of All Types

There is only one age group in the entire spectrum of life in which infectious disease is the leading killer. Children between the ages of 1 month and 1 year comprise that age group. This emphasizes the tremendous inroads that antibiotics and immunizations have made on infectious disease in this country. If one goes back 20 years, it becomes evident that infectious disease is the leading killer throughout most of the pediatric period. This is encouraging to those of us who have watched the changing pattern of medicine over the past quarter of a century. However, one cannot look at the chart objectively and not be a little embarrassed that there are still so many deaths from infectious disease in this 11-month period.

Further elaboration of this entry is warranted. We must mention the change in infant environment from the sterile intrauterine locale to the semisterile nursery, then hopefully to the clean home. In this way the infant is gradually introduced to unsanitary conditions, and with each new exposure he has the opportunity to develop his own immunity to replace that furnished by his mother. Certainly, any mother who has dedicated herself to raising this infant as prescribed in the preceding chapters will take good care of the baby. She will already have discussed this problem with her pediatrician. Standards for food preparation, linen laundry, and home environment will have been considered and be under control. Unfortunately, not all things are predictable and controllable. Infants become exposed to organisms to which they have limited immunity, and they become ill. It is at this point that medical care must intervene on behalf of the infant.

Of the 10,778 infants dying of infectious disease, we find that 5600 of these deaths were caused by pneumonia. Meningitis and encephalitis contributed another 1000 deaths. The next largest entry in this group is gastroenteritis or colitis, which also contributes nearly 1000 deaths. Various infections make up the remaining deaths.

I would like to see this number reduced to zero, as would every other physician. It is in this group that we feel we should be able to reduce mortality. From a practical standpoint we know that zero deaths from infectious disease is an impossibility, even though theoretically it appears feasible. To reduce further the mortality in this category will require a combined effort on the part of the family of the infant and the physician caring for the infant. If the infant is febrile, has difficulty breathing, assumes an unusual posture, or does not eat normally, try to arrive at an explanation. If the child's condition seems to be changing rapidly or if the change does not comport with any reasonable explanation, it is time to discuss the situation with the pediatrician. At this point the family shares the responsibility for the child's care with one more knowledgeable. His approach will depend upon his experience over the years and in the last few days—there are frequently local infectious epidemics that may explain the child's symptoms—as well as his knowledge of you and your baby.

The pediatrician may request X ray consultation. If the diagnosis is pneumonia, the radiologist tries to help by determining the extent of the disease and, if possible, by helping with its bacteriology. X ray is not generally helpful in determining what type of organism is causing the pneumonia. There are exceptions. Recently we had the opportunity radiographically to make the diagnosis of a staphylococcus pneumonia within the first few hours of symptoms. The treatment was well under way before the bacteriological confirmation was received. This may have been life-saving. If not, it certainly reduced the length of the hospitalization for that given infant.

So far we have said nothing concerning immunizations. This is such a well-established preventive medicine procedure that we assume that it is well under way during this time period. All pediatricians follow a routine immunization program. It includes immunization against whooping cough, diphtheria, polio, measles, tetanus, and in some instances smallpox. There have been recommendations that the smallpox immunization be deleted. This seems reasonable, since there has not been a case in the United States for several years, and there are times when for specific reasons smallpox immunizations should not be used. Immunization programs have done even more than antibiotics to reduce the infectious disease toll. They are a vital part of the preventive disease program. See the following chart for recommendations of the American Academy of Pediatrics.

Chart X

IMMUNIZE YOUR CHILD*

Measles, rubella, polio, whooping cough, diphtheria and tetanus are not just harmless childhood diseases. All of them can cripple or kill.

All are preventable. In order to be completely protected against diphtheria, tetanus and whooping cough (pertussis) your child needs a shot of the combination diphtheria-tetanus-pertussis (DTP) vaccine at two, four, six, and eighteen months and a booster when he goes to school.

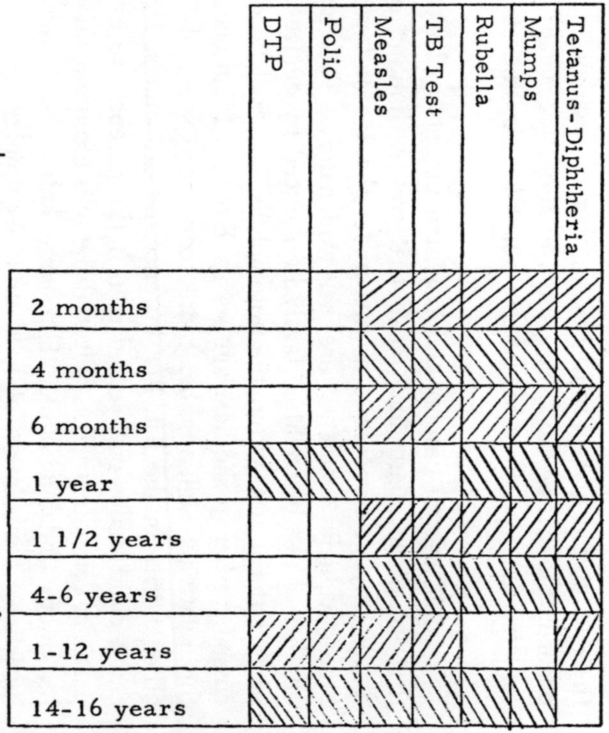

When he gets his DTP shots he should also get a drop of the oral polio vaccine.

After his first birthday your child should have a shot for measles, rubella and mumps. This also can be given in one combination shot. He should be tested for tuberculosis in his first year, and when he's 14 to 16 years make sure he gets his tetanus diphtheria booster shot.

*Recommended by The American Academy of Pediatrics

Published by the American Academy of Pediatrics.

Accidents

The pattern of accidents varies with age. The child prior to age one is just starting to walk. He certainly is not driving an automobile and he is not swimming. Accidents that occur in this period are very much the responsibility of the parents. For this reason we feel that it will be valuable to detail the accidents that occur in the first year of life. If we add those accidents that occur from the 28th day to the end of the first year to the number of accidents that occur in the first 28 days, we have a total of 2751. Chart IX explains the type of accidents that occur in this bracket.

I would ask all parents and potential parents to look at that list of accidents and recall that we are limiting our discussion at this point to infants under the age of 1 year. Motor vehicle accidents are self-explanatory. The total number of deaths could certainly be reduced by devices to protect the infant within the automobile. This will be discussed further in the next age series. Even so, I can accept this relatively high number more than I can some of the other entries in the list. For instance, 68 drownings! How can a child under one year drown if the parents are even partially competent? The falls and the fires are unfortunate, but more understandable. The large entry (620) under ingestion or inhalation of food or other objects is not acceptable and again reflects an area of carelessness on the part of the parents.

The classic example is the child who is eating peanuts or popcorn and for some reason chokes and aspirates a portion of the food particle into the lung. This is always a serious accident but, in most instances, should not prove fatal. First of all, let me say that this should be an entirely preventable accident, since children under the age of three have no business eating peanuts or popcorn. Peanuts are good protein, but should be given to children in the form of peanut butter rather than as the whole nut, which can so easily be aspirated by the infant who, at best, does a poor job of chewing his food. The child may have found the peanut on the floor; perhaps it was a bean or similar vegetable object. If the child coughs or chokes, a physician should be notified. Although the vegetable foreign body is not opaque to X ray, such a foreign body in the bronchus can be expected to produce characteristic X ray changes. Once its position is established, the foreign body can usually be removed through a bronchoscope. Needless to say, the younger the child, the more hazardous this procedure becomes. There should certainly be far less than 620 fatalities from such aspirations each year.

Unfortunately, the type of incident described above occurs to only part of the patients listed in this 620 deaths. It also includes ingestions of foodstuffs or other objects that result in fatality. Lead poisonings from eating paint chips are relatively few in number, but do occur in children under one year of age. Most of us are far more concerned about the child who ingests household poisons, particularly caustic chemicals used for cleaning drains or poisoning rodents or insects. The most pathetic of all accidents we encounter is the child whose esophagus has been destroyed by caustics, particularly the type used to clean drains. Untreated, the child would die of starvation because of inability to pass food from the mouth to the stomach. Even when gastrostomy is performed, and the patient is fed through a tube in the abdominal wall, he cannot swallow his own saliva and constantly drools. Dilation or reconstruction of the esophagus is a long and tedious process and is, at best, no more than a substitute for the real thing. I am certain that, if every new mother could make a tour through the wards of our children's hospitals and see some of the suffering and disability that occurs with accidental poisonings of this type, she would be so impressed that she would make her home a haven of safety. These deaths should be preventable. As the child starts to explore, as he should, discipline and guidance are critical. Discipline does not just mean spanking, but proper communication regarding dangerous places and objects.

Crib death is a real entity. There was a time when some of us felt that crib deaths were suffocation, and we were concerned that some might be homicide. With the accumulation of predeath data and more autopsy studies, crib death can generally be separated from homicide. No single mechanism of producing crib death is known. It is one of the real disasters of infancy. It occurs in young families, who invariably feel they have done something wrong. They are grief- and guilt-stricken. Autopsy studies fail to explain the death. We do know that infants breathe very poorly through their mouths; if for some reason the nose becomes occluded, the child may suffocate before he learns to mouth-breathe properly. We do know that colds or virus infections are common in these children. Therefore, crib death may occur in a young infant whose nose becomes occluded by any means at a time when he is still unable to roll over or to adjust. Dr. J. L. Caddell reports that magnesium deficiency is a cause of crib death. Others, such as Dr. Swift of Sheffield, England feel that there must be multiple causes of this entity. In the November 29, 1973 issue of *The New England Journal of Medicine*, a Philadelphia group presented evidence to show that the heart-conduction system in the crib-death infant was different from that of normal infants. After you read our Chapter XI, you will agree that there is logic in studying this system. The next issue of this same medical journal carried evidence suggesting that the conversion of fetal hemoglobin to adult hemoglobin may play an important role in crib death. Therefore, we must now admit there is no one complete explanation for this problem.

Our vital statistics data list only 522 deaths in this category. This is admittedly low, for it has been difficult for the attending physician to code this death properly. This is being changed. No doubt some of these deaths were called pneumonia or were placed in vague categories, to be discussed later. A national organization has been formed to raise funds to study crib death, or suddent infant death syndrome (S.I.D.S.), now the more popular term. A recent press release by this group stated that from 15,000 to 25,000 children die each year of this syndrome. Since this occurs almost exclusively in the 28-day to 1-year age group and since Chart VIII indicates that the total number of deaths in this age group was 20,901, we must conclude that this group was overreacting emotionally to the situation. More rational estimates of the incidence of crib death are in the 3000 to 5000 deaths-per-year range. We should have quite accurate figures in the next few years.

The largest number of accidental deaths are unexplained. It seems unusual that 807 infants under the age of one should have died by accident and still that type of accident be unknown. Keep this in mind as we discuss the next group of children.

Deaths From Ill-Defined Conditions and All Other Diseases

Between the 28th day of life and the end of the first year, the deaths of 2744 children are classified as caused by ill-defined symptoms, ill-defined conditions, and all other diseases. By going to a more detailed table, we are able to extract some groups of death attributable to disease we all recognize. The following list is informative:

Ill-defined symptoms and conditions	1937
All other diseases	807
Cystic fibrosis	179

Diseases of the adrenal gland	19
Thymic disease	35
Benign tumors	50

It is not out of place for us to question the accuracy of vital statistics data. Dr. J. F. Kurtzke, in his book entitled *Epidemiology of Cerebral Vascular Disease,* devotes an entire chapter to the validity of mortality data. The accuracy of such data is related directly to the number of autopsies made on the deaths that compose the data. There is no way of knowing how many autopsies were done on the children who died under 1 year of age. We do know that autopsies are frequently not performed in this age group, and that is probably the reason so many deaths fall into vague categories.

The diagnosis of death caused by thymic disease has been out of medical favor for at least 20 years. Most of us feel that the thymus gland does not cause death except when it is grossly invaded with a malignant disease. Even though the number of deaths attributed to thymic disease is relatively small (35), I am certain that in active children's hospitals other diagnoses would have been offered.

Cystic fibrosis has received considerable publicity in the last few years. This disease involves the secretory glands of different organs. The mucous glands of the lungs do not adequately clear the dirt and particles from the lung. Sweat glands tend to be altered to the point where considerable salt is lost from the body; this makes hot weather a dangerous time for children with this disability. The intestinal secretions from the newborn are thick and sticky and may produce genuine obstruction. These facts make cystic fibrosis a legitimate and evident cause of death in this age group.

Diseases of the adrenal gland are difficult to diagnose. These, too, result in a loss of salt, and children may die suddenly and mysteriously because of loss of electrolytes from the body. It is very reasonable to assume that some of the unexplained deaths may be attributed to adrenal disease. If the percentage of autopsies in our age group of interest increased, I am sure this diagnosis would have appeared more than 19 times.

A benign tumor that produces a fatality can hardly be classified as benign. However, we do have a paradox in terminology. When we speak of malignant tumors, we are referring to tumors that start in one location and spread to another, either by direct invasion, through the bloodstream or through the lymphatics. A tumor that arises at a single site and shows no inclination to spread is classified as benign. It is, therefore, possible for a benign tumor to be fatal. An example of this is a cyst in a critical area of the brain.

After we have extracted the deaths caused by cystic fibrosis, adrenal disease, thymus disease, and benign tumors, we still have 524 deaths in the "other diseases" category, and 1937 deaths that are specifically attributed to "ill-defined symptoms and conditions." Additional adrenal deaths may account for part of this number. Some of the deaths may actually be crib deaths. Unfortunately, some of these cases are homicides. No one really knows the number of homicides in infants, but it seems to be higher than the number actually given. It is easy to understand that the diagnosis of homicide is not popular, for it is an extremely difficult diagnosis to prove. The physician may be seeing a deceased infant for the first time. He is inclined to give the family the benefit of the doubt. This may be even more true if the physician has known the family for some time and feels that they are incapable of such a crime. The physician, therefore, uses what he feels to be his best judgment and puts the death into the vital statistics in one of the vague categories. Post-mortem examinations would be very helpful in improving our statistical data, although even a necropsy is not absolutely reliable in detecting infant homicide. Total body X rays should be included in infant post-mortems because there are fractures that are rather characteristic of infant abuse. Those of us who see cases of child abuse and recognize them as relatively frequent occurrences are most skeptical of death by "ill-defined symptoms." The number of child abuse cases per year is not known. At the Children's Mercy Hospital in Kansas City we see approximately 120 such cases a year. This probably represents less than one quarter of those that occur in our community of 1.5 million people. Dr. Kempe of the University of Colorado has estimated that there are as many as 60,000 abused children per year, or about 300 cases per million population. Of course, not all of these are fatal; any estimate of the number of fatalities on this basis would be a pure guess. Such homicide will be dealt with below.

Homicide

By adding the 117 homicides reported for the first 28 days of life to the 109 homicides reported from the 28th day to the end of the first year, we have a total of 226 homicides for the first year of life in our year of interest, 1967. As you have no doubt gathered from our discussion of accidents and deaths attributed to vague causes, we suspect that there are more homicides than the relatively small number listed. It seems that a fair argument can be offered for a number nearer 2000 rather than several hundred.

Child abuse is a highly publicized syndrome. Information concerning it has appeared on television documentaries, in the newspapers, and in books. There are many well-recognized authorities in this field. I would like to list two books that warrant study if you are interested in this entity. The first is entitled *Children in Jeopardy* by Dr. E. Elmer of the University of Pittsburgh School of Medicine, published by the University of Pittsburgh Press in 1967. The second book, by Dr. C. Henry Kempe and Ray E. Helfer, is entitled *Helping the Battered Child and Its Family,* published by J. B. Lippincott in 1972. Dr. Kempe is Chairman of the Department of Pediatrics at the University of Colorado and has been very active in this field for a number of years. Dr. Helfer is now at Michigan State University, but was formerly with Dr. Kempe at Denver. Another physician who deserves mention in this area is Dr. John Caffey, one of the pioneer pediatric radiologists in this country. During his many years at Baby's Hospital in New York he emphasized the X ray evidence of trauma on the infant skeleton and taught many of us to recognize this entity.

The reaction of the medical community to this syndrome has been a predictable one when one looks at it in historical context. Initially, most physicians were aghast and shocked, disbelieving that parents or other adults would abuse children to the point of death. After this initial shock had passed and it became apparent that this was a real situation, there was anger, a cry for punishment, and the passage of many laws. We now seem to be developing a more mature attitude toward this entity, and great effort is being placed on prevention of death to the child by vigorously treating the parent or parent substitute.

The highest incidence of this practice occurs to children under the age of two. However, no age group is immune until one reaches the mid-teens, and there have been reported cases of serious beatings and abuses even in early teen-age children. It has been stated that nearly 30 per cent of the children were somewhat abnormal prior to the abuse period. This raises concern over the possible role of the prevocative or the tyrannical child. Certainly, all of us recognize that the personalities of children differ. It has been estimated that some 5 to 10 per cent of infants are provocative and tyrannical. We know that most abused children come from families of the low socioeconomic group. One statistical series reports that 60 per cent of such families received government assistance during the year in which the abuse occurred. This syndrome nevertheless crosses all socioeconomic lines. Since it has occurred in families of professional people, including physicians and ministers, no group seems to be immune. A high percentage of parents who abuse children themselves were neglected or abused. It is also known that about one third of abused children are from fatherless homes. In most instances the abuser is the mother; however, a number of cases are reported where the abuse was perpetrated by the baby-sitter, a stepfather, the mother's boyfriend, or even a sibling.

A medical definition of the syndrome has been written by Dr. John Caffey; it is defined generally as the intentional or nonaccidental physical injury inflicted on infants and younger children. Usually this is done by distraught parents (90 per cent), less commonly by parent substitutes, or by anyone to whom infants may be exposed. The physical injury can occur in any form. It can include both trauma produced by fire and mechanical injury. The definition should also include abandonment, neglect, and exploitation, for these situations also occur. This entity has characterized society for many centuries. Certainly, those who have read the novels of Charles Dickens are well aware of the cruelties to which older children were subjected during his era. Infanticide may be an accepted practice in underdeveloped countries when food becomes scarce and parents feel it is more humane to eliminate the child than to see it suffer. Only rarely is this a motive that leads to infant abandonment in contemporary society. More commonly, the abuser does not know how to let the child grow and develop as a child. Parental demands are excessive; to survive, the child becomes adultlike early in life. There is usually a precipitating family crisis, but this crisis is only the tip of the iceberg—solving the immediate crisis may be important, but therapy must be directed at more than the precipitating crisis.

Roman law provided that fathers had absolute power over their childen, including the right to decide such matters as life and death, freedom, and slavery. The state protected this right of the father and regarded the offspring as the property of that parent. English law tended to follow the same line, except that it stipulated that fathers had a responsibility for support and protection of their children as well as control of their destiny. As time progressed, the responsibility of parents increased, and their dictatorial powers diminished. During the present century there has been increased concern over the inherent rights of children, on the basis of which laws for their protection have been passed.

It seems that we are now saying that the newborn baby has inherent rights and is an individual who belongs to his parents only so far as they maintain their responsibility for reasonable care and development. If the parents neglect the child or do not maintain an adequate home, the court then has the power to remove the child from that home, to act in its behalf, and place it in a foster home. These laws tend to reflect the evolution of a more sophisticated society. As I have tried to point out in previous chapters, having a child is a privilege. It should be so planned that this child has an ideal environment from the time of conception until he is an independent individual. The parent-child relationship is now one of stewardship, not ownership.

It is understandable that there will be problems in knowing when child abuse occurs. After all, a parent is expected to discipline his children. When does reasonable discipline end and child abuse begin? This certainly is a matter of judgment. However, the laws of all states now require that, whenever child abuse is suspected, it is to be reported to the proper officials. This means that the physician is obligated to report such cases. Most children's hospitals have set up committees to review cases before calling on the assistance of the courts. This is but another step in our attempt to be less emotional and more helpful in this very serious situation.

The disposition of such cases is dependent upon the findings in the case. The reaction of the person guilty of abusing the child is extremely important. One must evaluate whether this abuse will recur or if this was a one-time affair. The willingness of the abuser to seek therapeutic aid through some form of counseling is important. Under some circumstances, it is possible to return the child to the family providing that they keep in contact with the responsible physician or counseling group. In other instances it is necessary for the protection of the child that he be separated from the family, at least during the time the family is seeking aid and counsel. When substantial improvement has been observed or adequate insight is gained into the problem, the child may then be returned to the family. On other occasions, particularly where there is evidence that child abuse in the family has been chronic or repetitive, it is necessary to disassociate the infant from the family permanently. Some 15 years ago we felt that an abused child returned to his home environment had a 50 per cent mortality rate. We implied that, if we made the diagnosis of child abuse and confronted the parents, but did nothing to correct the situation except return the child to his home, the child would probably be subject to more hostility than before. I do not know where the 50 per cent figure for mortality arose. It was apparently more emotional than scientific, for most of the information reported now implies that the figure is more nearly 10 per cent. Even this is dangerous. A rule in every children's institution is to not return an abused child to the same environment unless some active measures have been taken in regard to improving that environment.

To prevent homicide would seem impossible. However, we have implied in the previous paragraphs that the diagnosis of child abuse can be made in less than fatal instances. Preventive measures need to be reemphasized. If there is any question, the child should be placed in a foster home, either on a temporary or permanent basis. To those of us who have seen these problems, it is perfectly apparent that some parents are too stupid to raise children. Their offspring are neglected, uncared for, and malnourished. Other parents are psychotic and dangerous to their infants. Fortunately, these two groups make up a minority. It seems that most parents who have by misfortune been driven to child abuse are salvageable by treatment, so that the parents and children can be reunited. Since we are not certain how many homicides occur as a result of child abuse, it would be futile to estimate how many homicides might be prevented.

Tolerance and guidance must be offered to mothers or abusing parents who seem to be correctable. A mother may find it difficult to be with a child 24 hours a day even when a father is present and when there are no economic problems. Under less than an ideal arrangement, the tensions on the mother mount. There is apparently no way in which this responsibility can be abdicated; however, options and help must be made available through family, friends or, if need be, such impersonal sources as day-care units or other government agencies.

There is good evidence to show that there is hope of preventing homicide in children. Unfortunately, the preventive measures, while very real, are somewhat vague. Specialists such as Dr. Ray E. Helfer are teaching pediatricians by lecture and consultation to recognize parents who are potentially dangerous to children before trouble arises. This is true preventive medicine and offers real hope.

Looking to the Future

Basically this entire discussion has looked to the future. We have stated that the planning of a pregnancy should start a year prior to conception. Now, as we approach the end of our discussion involving the first year of life, we need to look seriously at events in later life that might be modified by habits and training at this early age. We now want to plan the child's future so that he will achieve maximum intellectual growth and development and so that his physical health will be of such a quality that the incidence of disease will be minimized.

The fundamentals of infant nutrition have changed very little over the years. However, because of the high adult death rate from coronary heart disease and because we know that changes that occur in the pediatric period tend to predispose to coronary heart disease, we are making some very careful reevalutions of infant feeding. Infant feeding and its relationship to adult coronary heart disease have been carefully studied by a joint commission of the American Academy of Pediatrics and the American Heart Association. As might be expected, the heart group recommended changes in infant feeding, while the American Academy of Pediatrics felt that any dramatic change in infant nutrition might result in complications worse than the heart problem for which we were seeking a solution. Despite what may seem an impasse, I am certain that both groups gained additional information from their discussions and that the patient will be the beneficiary. For instance, the pediatricians made the point that a certain amount of fat in the diet of infants is very necessary for adequate formation of skin and brain and the absorption of fat-soluble vitamins. Normal development of brain and skin must be just as important as the possible later heart problem. On the other hand, it was pointed out by the Heart Association that these necessary fats can be provided without giving the infant excessive amounts of fat, particularly animal fat, thereby offering some qualitative improvement in the type of fat itself. It would seem that the pediatricians have been forcefully informed that some of our traditional American foods must be either eliminated, or sharply curtailed, if adult life is to be full, active, and safe.

Most physicians agree that the ideal starting food for the infant is breast milk. However, we all know that this is not critical and that there are many substitutes. Cow's milk formulas can be worked out in a very satisfactory and economical manner. Commercial infant feeding formulas are more expensive, but offer a closer approximation to breast milk than the standard cow's milk formulas. The ratio of saturated fatty acids to polyunsaturated fatty acids in breast milk and in most commercial formulas is approximately one to one. However, cow's milk contains twice as much saturated fatty acid as unsaturated. Our cardiology friends would like to see twice as much polyunsaturated fat as saturated. The cholesterol level also tends to be higher in the cow's milk formulas. This disadvantage of cow's milk can be corrected by using part nonfat milk and by additional dilution. With a little care and calculation adequate diets can be arranged to embody all of the needed nutritional elements at relatively low cost. It may not be possible or ideal to eliminate cholesterol and to have two parts of polyunsaturated fatty acids to one part saturated fatty acids in the same formula; still, with some thought, reasonable ratios and levels can be maintained. Clinical trials now underway look encouraging.

Your pediatrician or his assistant will advise the proper time for the addition of vegetables and cereal. The addition of fruits to the diet is generally delayed in hopes that the infant will accept cereals and vegetables before being introduced to the sweet taste of fruits. Vitamin supplements will be given, and iron supplements may be used, depending upon the growth, development, and appearance of the child. At this time parents should be reminded that salting to adult tastes is not necessary for children. Modest or no salting should be the rule. The addition of egg yolk to the diet has been a favorite practice of pediatricians and nutritionists for many years. Elimination or reduction of this component is another way of reducing cholesterol exposure. Other sources of fat calories may be required, and iron supplements may be indispensable at this point. Most of us feel that no adult, much less a 12-pound infant should have one egg yolk per day. In case you do not know, egg yolks contain 1500 milligrams of cholesterol per 100 grams of egg yolk. Although the content depends on the size of the egg, each egg yolk contains approximately 240 milligrams of cholesterol. The American Heart Association suggests that 300 milligrams be the total adult daily intake of cholesterol. Because of these high levels of cholesterol, those of us who are interested in preventive medicine strongly advocate that the use of egg yolk in infant diet supplement be reduced or the diet modified in such a way that total cholesterol content will be more reasonable. No one has ever seen a disease recognizable as cholesterol deficiency. Rigid fat restriction is not advocated at this age. We will recommend reduced fat intake after one year, but this will not be a severe restriction—only an attempt to lower what we now consider the excessive fat ingestion of all American children.

In addition to the quality of food, the quantity given the infant is also under scrutiny. For many years we have operated on the concept of minimum daily requirements of given vitamins or food elements. Such a concept tended toward overfeeding, for it said to the physician or the mother, "This is the least amount of these elements your baby needs" and implied, "The more he gets of these things, the better." Obviously, this is an untrue statement. Fat babies are not healthy babies any more than fat adults are healthy adults. Nutritionists are now in the process of examining food requirements with the idea of developing maximum quantities that should be consumed. At the same time, another look should be taken at the minimum daily requirements, since many of these are probably well above the true minimum standards required by infants or, for that matter, even adults. A good general rule is "Don't stuff the baby." The "clean-up-your-plate" philosophy has no doubt contributed a great deal to our problem of obesity. It has been shown that the number of fat cells a person will have is determined by the time he reaches one year of age. We may not be able to prevent obesity in adults by preventing it in children, but there is evidence that implies that nonfat babies have less trouble with obesity in later years than do children who are fat at the end of the first year of life.

At this point, we need to discuss malnutrition more thoroughly. If a baby is born with a low birth weight for his gestation age, we assume that there has been some malnourishment *in utero.* This may possibly have been caused by faulty maternal nutrition, maternal illness, or any number of other reasons that we have mentioned. However, a significant number of these low-birth-weight infants are the result of placental abnormalities. The placenta is the vascular organ that connects the baby and the mother. If the placenta is small or fails to function normally, the fetus will not be adequately nourished. Unfortunately, we know of no way in which placental function can be predicted during pregnancy, and we know of no way in which abnormal function of the placenta can either be prevented or treated.

As a result of this, we occasionally have low birth weight for gestation-age infants born despite all the precautions that the physician and mother can take. The degree of handicap this infant suffers depends upon the degree to which his size has been reduced during the gestational period. The number of brain and lung cells have been diminished because of this intrauterine malnutrition. However, if this infant is a full-term baby and if his weight is in the area of 5 pounds, his handicaps generally can be overcome by special care and feeding during his first six months of life. This group of infants is a high-risk, but salvageable, group. On the other hand, if malnutrition occurred *in utero* and is complicated by poor feeding after birth, the problem of growth and mental retardation is compounded. The number of brain cells, like the number of fat cells, is determined by the end of the first year of life. Therefore, the physical development necessary for normal mental growth and development takes place *in utero* and during the first year of life. Since brain cells contain relatively high quantities of fat, you will understand why the American Academy of Pediatrics has not wholeheartedly adopted a fat restriction diet for infants and small children.

In our discussions of physical growth and development, we have implied that normal growth is necessary for mental and intellectual development. The principles of intellectual development are surprisingly similar to those of physical development. If one is to be intelligent and mentally active, one must be in a stimulating environment and receive those stimuli that are necessary to intellectual growth. Just as muscles grow and become more efficient with exercise, so the brain grows and becomes more efficient in a stimulating environment. Here again, we must not wait until the child is ready for school and assume that all of this learning will take place in those hallowed halls. Preschool programs have been set up in a number of localities in an attempt to improve the subsequent performance of children in school. This is undoubtedly a step in the right direction. However, every mother must be made aware of the fact that a stimulating environment must begin at home, and that the stimulus should be added to the pattern of life at a very early age. Of course, we do not imply that the mother should read Shakespeare to the infant. The child needs to be introduced gradually to his environment. This includes household objects, toys, and articles of various shapes and sizes. Each item becomes a new discovery. As soon as the child can crawl, he has another means of exploring. This should be encouraged. Sharp objects and items that might be swallowed or inhaled should be kept away from the exploration area. It also goes without saying that stairways and objects that can be pulled over represent hazards to our new explorer and should be removed from the area of his exploration. The same should be said for fireplaces and stoves; it is here that the child is taught about danger and assured that discipline is a form of love and protection.

To summarize our experience with this ideal child's first year of life, we must conclude: 1. Don't bring him into the world until he is at full term. 2. Feed him well and adequately, but do not overfeed him. 3. Love and stimulate the child frequently, but in doing so remember that he must be protected from those things that are so dangerous to children, mainly infections and accidents.

VII. The Beginnings of Emancipation
Ages 1 Through 4

The Bureau of Vital Statistics defines this age as the period of time from the child's first birthday up to his fifth birthday. This age group enjoys a very significant 26-fold decrease in the mortality rate compared to the first year. This striking decrease in mortality rate should be taken as an indication of the great dangers of the first year of life rather than of the relative safety of the next four years. This period offers to parents a great opportunity to discipline the child in the proper eating habits and to develop the sense of safety that is so greatly needed in the ensuing decades. Chart XI summarizes the mortality statistics for this segment of our population.

You will note that, instead of reporting the actual numbers of deaths in each category, we are using death rate statistics. This is based on the number of deaths per 100,000 population in this age group. I have some reservation in using death rate statistics rather than raw data; however, virtually all medical and statistical data are presented in terms of deaths per 100,000 rather than in actual numbers. There will be occasions when actual numbers will be used.

For those more interested in actual numbers than in death rates, the total population in the 1 through 4 age group in 1967 was 15,652,000. Therefore, with the rates per 100,000 given, the raw numbers can be generated by simply multiplying the number given as death rate by 156.5. Another advantage of using death rate statistics rather than actual numbers is that we are comparing smaller numbers, and most of us can compare one- or two-digit numbers more easily than four- and five-digit numbers.

The chart presents few surprises. You should notice promptly that we now have a new leading cause of death. Even at this tender age, accidents have become the leading killer. More than a third of all deaths in the age group are accidental. Accidents are the leading cause of death in this age group in part because of our better control of infectious disease. Ten-year trends indicate that infectious disease has been declining as a killer, while accidental deaths are on the increase.

We shall not detail the types of accidents that produce death in this category. I will mention that the leading cause of death from accidents was the motor vehicle, followed by fire and drowning.

Infectious disease is the second most common cause of death in this age group. The distribution of deaths among the infectious diseases is virtually the same as in the last age group. Pneumonia is by far the most common cause of death by infection. Infection of the central nervous system ranks second; this includes both meningitis and encephalitis. Other than these, infections are a relatively rare cause of death.

Congenital heart disease is the most common fatal congenital anomaly in this age distribution; congenital defects in the central nervous system are next in order. Over the last ten years (see Appendix, Chart I), one is impressed by the decreasing incidence of congenital anomalies as a cause of death. These figures represent all age groups. In 1958, 12.4 deaths per 100,000 were caused by congenital anomalies; in 1967 this had fallen to 8.8 deaths per 100,000. This represents a very significant decrease in deaths from this cause. The reasons for the decrease are twofold. First, many of the very severe congenital anomalies such as those attributable to rubella infection of the mother are being prevented. Second, a number of congenital disorders are being treated surgically with reasonable success. There is no doubt that the number of children dying of congenital heart disease is decreasing because of the development of very fine surgical and anesthetic techniques in this area. It is encouraging to see an area in which both prevention and treatment are lowering the overall mortality.

We discussed homicide at some length in the last section. Very little can be added here. I am still inclined to feel that the given incidence of 1 per 100,000 in this age group is low. However, since there are fewer "vague" deaths in this age group, the hidden homicides are much more difficult to find. Some of the accidents may have been homicides. Again, this is a particularly difficult statement to verify.

Malignancy in children of this age group warrants some additional discussion. You will note that malignancy has moved into fourth place as a cause of death. It will tend to move up as our age groups become older. Most of us think of malignancy as a disease of the elderly. However, as you see here, this is not entirely the case. By going back to the raw data in our general mortality statistics, the following list is offered for the breakdown of deaths caused by malignancy in this age group.

Leukemia and lymphoma	705
Brain and nervous tissue	319
Malignancy of urinary tract	99
Malignancy of digestive tract (including the liver)	39
Other less common and unlisted sites of origin	121
Total	1283

Cancer is a very complicated disease. Basically, the cells multiply and grow out of control. The nature of the cells that grow out of control is dependent upon the primary cell, or the cell of origin, of the malignancy. For this reason we refer to a primary cancer of a given organ to imply that this is the type of cell that started growing out of control. The malignancy that arises from brain cells may follow an entirely different course than one that arises in the cells that make up the liver. Therefore, there are as many different kinds of cancer as there are different types of cells in the human body. This very simplified explanation of malignancy is offered only to make the previous chart more understandable. When we refer to lymphomas and leukemia, we are saying that the cancer cells had their origin in lymphatic tissue, lymph glands, or the cells that make up the blood-forming tissues. When we refer to malignancy of the urinary tract as the site of origin, it could be either in the bladder, the kidney or the ureters.

We know that the types of malignancies change a great deal as the years advance. You will note that there are no cancers of the lung listed in this category, yet when we reach older age groups it will become a very common type of malignancy. Except for the brain tumors, most of the malignancies in children are present as masses. These masses may actually be seen or may be felt on careful examination. This statement is made only to point up the importance of any mass that appears in a youngster. Of course, not all masses are malignant, but with the appearance of any mass some explanation for its presence needs to be determined.

As one interested in preventive medicine, at this point in time we have nothing to offer to the parent or the child as a technique for preventing these malignant tumors. As a physician who is involved in the diagnosis and treatment of disease, I can be somewhat more encouraging. Improved surgery, radiation therapy, and chemotherapy are reducing the incidence of death from malignant disease. Unfortunately, the rate of improvement is much less dramatic than we would like, but on some types of nervous tissue tumor (neuroblastoma) and on certain types of kidney tumors (Wilms' Tumor) there are definite statistical improvements. The leukemias are showing considerably improved survival time, although most of us are still rather cautious about speaking of cures in this area. Modest optimism is offered in this disease.

Accident Prevention

As Chart XI indicated, the leading cause of death in this age group is accidents. The leading killer among the accidents is the motor vehicle. For these reasons it seems pertinent to discuss a few principles of accident prevention for small children. It is a common sight when driving about suburbia to see a mother with several children in her car; the children are standing or moving freely about the front or back seats of the vehicle. Unstable legs and a relatively high center of gravity make a fall associated with a sudden stop a virtual certainty. No farmer would be so careless about taking his eggs to market. Any such valuable and breakable item would be securely fastened to the automobile so that acceleration or deceleration would not result in breakage. Yet our child, a very breakable item and hopefully worth more than a crate of eggs, enjoys no such protection. We all know adults do not use seat belts as often as they should. It is a human frailty to feel that safety measures are unnecessary. In addition to this frailty, children tend to be unhappy when confined, and expressions of this unhappiness can make for a nervous driver. Compounding the problem further is the relative lack of suitable restraining devices for children in automobiles. Certainly, the conventional shoulder and lap belts used for adults are not usable in the same manner for small children. The American Academy of Pediatrics has approved a certain number of child-fixation devices for use in automobiles. *Consumer Reports* has also tested and reported on a number of these devices. These are marketed by Ford, General Motors, Sears, and a few other companies. Any device is better than nothing, but some tend to be better than others.

For children of 25 to 50 pounds, the shield-type seat "Tot Guard" by Ford is recommended. For children over 50 pounds, an adult belt can be used, but shoulder harness crosses too near the neck to warrant its use. When a child is more than 55 inches tall, he may use both seat and shoulder harnesses.

Beware of poorly designed restraints, especially those that merely hook over the back of the seat. Some examples of approved child fixation devices are shown in Chart XII In addition, the following general precautions are suggested. The back seat is generally safer than the front seat. Therefore, as a general rule, children should be kept in the back. If there are rear doors they should be kept locked. This is one advantage of the two-door automobile for a young family. Place the child in the back seat in a safety or restraining device and you have done about all that can be offered for the child at this point. If the child is still in an infant basket or basinette, the housing can be fixed to the back seat by a seat belt. The long axis of the basinette should be directed along the long axis of the car and strong soft netting placed over the top to keep the child from being thrown forward in the event of sudden stops. The feet should be directed toward the front seat. A child on the mother's lap, even if the mother is wearing a seat belt, is very dangerous because of the short distance from the baby to the dash or seat ahead. From here on, the safety of the child is in the hands of the driver of this automobile and the drivers of other automobiles in our concrete sea.

Accidental poisoning, one of the real perils of toddlers, took 310 lives in our 1-through-4 age group in 1967. A round figure for deaths in the entire pediatric age group from accidental poisoning is 500. It is apparent that most accidental poisonings occur under the age of six. This is the age of the toddler, the curious infant, the exploring child, and the child whose intellectual growth we have encouraged you to stimulate. Three hundred and ten deaths in one age group as we have defined it here is not a large number. However, a low percentage of accidental poisonings is fatal. It is estimated that for each fatality from poisoning, there are at least 1000 children who are poisoned and recover. This high recovery rate is very gratifying and implies a job well done by people in the emergency rooms and in poison centers. However, as with so many illnesses, the poisoned child would have been better off had this accident not occurred.

It is not our intent to discuss all possible accidents to children and thus write a treatise on accident prevention. While accidental deaths certainly should be avoided, I accept the fact that there is no way of preventing all accidents. It is our hope to develop an attitude on the part of the parent and the child that will lead to the self-preservation and discipline that are so necessary to prevent accidents at all ages. Several general statistics are of some interest. Over three fourths of accidental poisonings occur in children under the age of five. By far the most common poisons to which children are exposed are common household products. Drugs of the "medicine cabinet" type are responsible for at least 50 per cent of the poisonings. Aspirin is the most common household drug; furniture polish, kerosene, vitamins, iron, diet pills, perfumes, turpentine, rubbing alcohol, paint, and as previously mentioned, the very corrosive drain cleaner compounds all seem to be fair game for the toddling youngster. Over 40 per cent of all poisonings occur in the kitchen. Twenty-one per cent occur in the bathroom; these are the common places where the dangerous items are stored.

If the child can see the medicine or toxic material, and

if it is brightly colored and in a clear bottle, he naturally feels that this is candy or something that he should explore. To a child, exploring means tasting and eating as well as seeing and touching. Therefore, the first rule in terms of poison prevention should be to keep all such compounds out of the sight of the child. Storage places for medicines and dangerous compounds should be either locked or stored at an inaccessible height. I remind you that it is easy to underestimate the child and his ability to climb to high places. Chairs, cupboards, toilet bowls, sinks all serve as ladders for our would-be explorer.

Children are great imitators. If they see a parent taking medication, they feel that this is something they should try. Recently we were reminded of this at the Children's Hospital. A three-year-old boy had seen his father attempt to siphon gasoline from a tank. This looked like fun, so the child tried it. Unfortunately, he was quite successful, and he is now in the hospital with rather extensive pneumonia produced by the hydrocarbons in the gasoline. I have no doubt that he will recover, but here again is an excellent example of "baby see, baby do."

The Federal government is taking steps to help in this area. The safety packaging act of 1970 will by 1974 require packaging to meet certain standards. Many of these containers were reported in *The Journal of Pediatrics* of October 1971 by a group of pediatricians and family practice physicians from the University of Utah. These reports will be extremely valuable to drug companies and to the government. Their studies seem to imply that the pressure release cap is the most effective in keeping children from the contents of the bottle. Other types of dispensers that individually package a given dosage of a drug also represent an improvement, since each dose must be unwrapped by the child. In this way the child ingests the drug more slowly and is more apt to be found by the parent before a lethal quantity can be consumed.

Here again we have an example of a significant medical problem being approached by various groups. The government is making regulations; the drug companies are anxious to comply. Physicians and those interested in preventive medicine will issue every type of warning. However, it all boils down to the responsibility of the family, which must see to it that poisonous compounds are not readily available, that safety packages are used, and that the infant is properly instructed and disciplined in the area of poison prevention.

Looking Ahead

There should be no risk at this point in substituting skim milk for whole milk. If one must have a spread on bread, peanut butter, honey, jelly, or both certainly represent a considerable reduction in cholesterol intake compared to butter, but not in calories. There is little reason for a child in this age group to have butter; of course, the same may be said of all age groups. If prejudice demands a yellow spread on bread, certainly the corn oil margarines offer considerable savings in cholesterol intake and represent a better balance between saturated and unsaturated fatty acids than butter.

Blood cholesterol levels have not been routinely done in children. However, as our concern over the high mortality rate from coronary heart disease increases, more cholesterol determinations will be done on children. High blood levels of fatty substances can be identified and classified. In this way high-risk persons, even infants and children, can be identified. Appropriate dietary restrictions can be imposed; the simple restrictions we have listed here may be more than adequate for most children, but some may require severe restrictions, including carbohydrate, especially sugars to keep the blood level of fats within an acceptable range.

The statements previously made in regard to overfeeding still hold true in the current age. One of the most important things the pediatrician or his assistant does when the child visits his office is to record the child's height and weight. Thus, growth and development can be measured and compared with normal standards. This offers an excellent check on the child's nutritional habits. In addition, it serves as an early warning sign in case of disease.

Other substances that could logically be reduced in amount from the usual diet with more benefit than harm include ice cream, desserts high in fat content and, of course, egg yolks, which we have previously mentioned. Everyone realizes that ice cream is a national staple in the diet of children. I am sure that its total elimination would be impossible and possibly not desirable. However, it certainly should not make up the large portion of the childhood diet that it now seems to provide. A real contribution to the American diet would be the development of a low-fat, polyunsaturated, cholesterol-free, and tasty ice cream. This may be developed. Standard Brands now is marketing an egg substitute, "Egg Beaters," which is cholesterol-free. It seems very satisfactory. Time will tell how well it will be accepted.

To this point we have said nothing about meat in the diet, yet everyone must know that meat is another source of cholesterol. Suffice it to say that meat should be served as lean as possible and should be broiled, boiled, or baked rather than fried. These points would seem to offer no difficulty to a child, and for that matter would offer very minimal changes so far as adults are concerned. These changes, however, would result in a considerable saving in cholesterol intake.

Again, we are looking at the overall problem and seriously listening to both the adult cardiologist and the pediatrician; knowing that all of us have the patient's best interest at heart, there seems to be little doubt that the patient will benefit.

VIII. The Decade of Discipline
Ages 5 Through 14

We have now reached a place where we can discuss as a block those children 5 to 14, inclusive. The mortality rate has dropped to the lowest figures they will reach at any time during their lives. Comparing Chart XIII with Chart XI (see Appendix) for the one-to-four-year-old infant, we can see that the mortality rates have dropped in every category, with the exception of those listed diseases that are generally regarded as characteristic of adults.

It is immediately obvious that accidents are still the leading cause of death in the current age group. Even so, the accident death rate has fallen approximately 40 per cent from the figure given for the earlier age. Even malignant disease has dropped from an incidence of 9.7 per 100,000 to 6.6. We can attribute this to the reduced number of leukemia and kidney tumor patients in this age group. Birth defects are also taking fewer lives now; this could be anticipated. The incidence of deaths from infectious disease also shows a precipitous drop; it is only about one-fourth as high as it was in the age-1-to-4 group.

Two new categories have been listed, although both of them are as yet very small. Both will increase in subsequent sections. Suicide is now a cause of death for the first time. The year 1967 records no suicides under the age of 9; however, there were 121 suicides between the ages of 10 and 14. The other category we list for the first time is coronary heart disease. Seven of our 27 patients were between the ages of 5 and 9, the other 20 between 10 and 14. There are some congenital anomalies that occur in the coronary arteries that predispose to early death; however, our mortality tables specifically list these as noncongenital lesions. One may well question the accuracy of the coding, but it is a well-known fact that coronary heart disease does affect young people; it seems that this is becoming more and more the case. Even knowing the high incidence of coronary heart disease and its ever-increasing prevalence, I find it difficult to accept 7 cases 9 years of age or younger. Despite our own prejudice, we will let the charts reflect the mortality rates. In searching for deaths that might be deferred, the age group 5 through 14 offers a relatively poor yield. The mortality rate of 41.4 per 100,000 is excellent. It is sad that all age groups cannot be equally fortunate. In 1967 the two five-year divisions of our population having the largest number of people were the groups age 5 through 9 and 10 through 14, respectively. There were 20,910,000 persons age 5 through 9, and there were 19,885,000 in the age group 10 through 14. This means that in the group we are now evaluating there were actually 40,795,000 people. This age group, therefore, represents not only the safest but the largest group we will be discussing. The most populous age group will change from year to year, depending upon the birth rate. The numbers given here reflect the high birth rates of the mid and late 50's.

Although accidents are the leading cause of death in our current age group, it has been noted that they are causing fewer deaths per 100,000 than they did in the one-to-four age group. I was surprised to find that this was true of most major types of accidents. There was a falling death rate in motor vehicle accidents, poisonings, falls, fires, explosions, and even drowning, compared to the younger age group. There were a few types of accidents that did have an increased mortality rate in the current age group. These included accidental death by firearms, death by electrocution, and a very slight increase in the death rate from water transportation accidents. The only explanation I can offer for the falling accidental death rate in car accidents has to do with the child's developing anatomy. Certainly, as the child ages, the skull is thicker and serious head injuries require a greater force than in the younger child. Another explanation may be that the children in this age group are more inclined to ride in the back seat and remain seated, while the very young child is more apt to be in front with the parent. I have no statistics to that effect; it only seems logical. I certainly believe that restraining devices for this age group are just as important as for the toddler. However, children in this age group tend to outgrow the fixation devices mentioned earlier; as they grow larger, adult lap belts and shoulder straps can be used with only minimal modifications.

In the 5-through-14 age group in 1967 there were 508 accidental deaths by firearms. I realize that firearm legislation is a very controversial subject. Even if there were no other deaths in younger or older age groups, it would seem that 508 children in this category are needless sacrifices for whatever pleasures adults may derive from guns. Any parent who is conscientious enough to follow our instructions in regard to avoiding poisonings in the earlier age group will either not have a gun in the house or will have it secured in such a way that even a 14-year-old cannot get it without the aid of his parent. Once again, safety around the home, in the automobile, and in virtually everything that we do must become a habit. Carelessness and additional risks are incompatible with the way of life that I am insisting upon here.

Accident Prevention

In the age group now under discussion, the child starts to school. For the first time we have a transportation problem that may not involve the family directly. Certainly, a majority of American schoolchildren are not taken to school by their parents. Some walk if they are fortunate enough to live close to the school, others may ride bicycles, and still others will be transported by the conventional school bus. There is no perfectly safe way of moving from home to school and back. Of course, this statement need not be limited to the schoolchild and his transportation problems, but is true of all of us. Young parents find the introduction of the child to the outside world and its hazards in transportation difficult.

For the child who walks to school, instruction on crossing the streets and observation of traffic hazards should be given by the parent and follow-up supervision and protection furnished by the police or school authorities. It seems that children are rarely injured going to and from school, since they usually move in groups, and motorists are quite aware of their presence. It is the child at play who darts out between cars in the middle of the street who is too frequently a victim of the oncoming automobile.

Bicycles are one of the real pleasures of childhood. In addition to the benefits of physical conditioning and the pleasures of their use, they offer an excellent mode of transportation. Bicycling to school is common, particularly in cities where streets are not congested. Deaths from bicycle accidents are relatively low. However, significant injury from bicycles is another matter. It has been estimated that there are 120,000 fractures and 60,000 contusions each year from bicycle accidents. This must be classed as a significant number; however, it represents only about one half of the children seriously injured in automobile accidents. There is no way of estimating the number of cuts, bruises, and other injuries that result in emergency room visits related to bicycle accidents. Dr. Julian Waller, reporting from the Vermont School of Medicine in *The Journal of Pediatrics* in June 1971, found in a school survey in his community that 2 per cent of bicycle owners are involved in significant accidents each year. Riding double and borrowing someone else's bicycle were the factors that seem predominantly to increase the risk. We are not implying that bicycles should be avoided, but it does seem pertinent to point out that they create a risk and that the child should attain a certain amount of skill before riding in the street or using the machine as his routine means of transportation to school.

The American school bus has been acclaimed as the safest form of passenger transportation in the world today. In 1967 the National Safety Council reported that 50 children were killed and 3800 injured in school buses. This was among 16.5 million pupils riding to and from school each day. This certainly appears to be an excellent safety record when compared to most other forms of transportation. Commercial airlines and buses alone have a better safety record. School buses do have a number of very favorable features. All of us accord the school bus respect. They are conspicuous in their size and color. It also seems unlikely that school buses would have the same driver intoxication problems as most other motor-driven vehicles. In addition, if an accident does occur, the size of the bus is an inherent safety factor. Despite these features, there are a number of problems. One of the most obvious is the fact that frequently the driver will be the only adult on the bus; therefore, he or she is burdened not only with the transportation, but with the discipline of the children. Most school buses have a rather "hostile" interior, with many hard metallic margins on the seats and body frame. Seat belts are frequently not installed or poorly installed and, even if available, may not be used in the absence of adult monitoring. Standing in school buses certainly should be prohibited. Again, this is difficult to enforce if the driver is the only adult on board. Most states require little in the way of qualifications for drivers. In fact, 17 states permit school buses to be driven by 16- and 17-year-olds. Fourteen states have a minimum age of 18 through 20. Only 19 states require that drivers be at least 21 years of age.

Government legislation in the area of standard regulations for school busing is in prospect and certainly seems to be required. Such regulations should include driver qualifications and education, as well as the safety construction of and devices on the school bus.

Health Activities

The years 5 through 14 are very active years and indeed a period of great change. It is at this time that the child is introduced to school, which should be nothing more than a new intellectual stimulus. It is at this time in his life that he is introduced to physical activity of a competitive type. Physical activity is very much to be encouraged in children. I do not wish to imply that all children should participate in the same sport with the same degree of vigor. There are certain children who obviously should be protected from the physical contact sports. Not all children should play football. Swimming, tennis, and bicycling have a great deal to offer in physical development and may be much more pleasurable to a given youngster than the more vigorous and dangerous contact sports. If one has any interest in sports, it is apparent that records are continuously being broken and that our young athletes are stronger, faster, and more agile than were the athletes of the previous decade. Part of these benefits are derived from the better health and nutrition of the athlete during his childhood years. In addition, early training plays an important role in his growth and development. The converse of this is also true, since it has been shown that athletic ability is related to early maturation.

It is certainly not our desire to make athletes of all youngsters. However, investigators have pointed out that one of the major problems in our adult population is our sedentary life. The enthusiasm of youth for athletic endeavors and physical sports certainly can do a great deal to avoid complacency and a sedentary existence in later years. Mr. Russel Sneedon of the Amateur Athletic Union in a letter to the editor of *The Journal of the American Medical Association* stated that, in general, the basis for physical fitness in adults is their physical fitness during their youth. It would seem that, if one can encourage young adults and children to enjoy physical activity, they are more apt to remain participants as adults. The natural energy level in children tends to be high; this is particularly true until puberty. It is important that the child's growth and development be observed and recorded through these critical years. This implies a continuing study, not just one-time measurements. Before any child participates in an athletic program, he should be examined by a physician and his growth and development evaluated. It must be remembered that the child will not only burn up energy in his athletic endeavors, but also will be using more calories for his growth and development than a nongrowing adult. Overzealous youngsters should be encouraged to moderation. Less vigorous youngsters should be encouraged to find endeavors they enjoy.

There are significant criticisms of such organized sports as Little League Baseball and similar football programs. They tend to be excessively competitive for children and parents. A few youngsters enjoy this type of competition, others may become so discouraged that in the future they will avoid all types of sports. This is unfortunate. We must also point out that baseball and football are not good sports for physical conditioning; they do little to improve heart function. Therefore, if a child is to participate in such programs, he should also engage in some activity that will make him physically fit for such events and improve his heart for later years. These activities must be such persistent forms of exercise as hiking, bicycling, swimming, or distance running.

In each of our previous sections we have discussed diet. It is no less important here. In general, our theme has been to avoid excess calories and to keep the total fat load as low as reasonably possible. We have also attempted to reduce the cholesterol level by eliminating those foods that are particularly high in cholesterol and hopefully substituting fats that are high in the polyunsaturated portions rather than in the saturated fatty acids. This becomes more difficult as the child becomes older. In this decade some important groundwork can be laid. The youngster is by now well accustomed to skim milk and would actually find whole milk unsatisfactory. Milk is good food to growing children, but milk is better without the fat than with it. It should be mentioned that man is the only animal that continues to consume milk after weaning. There may be a lesson in nature. The problems that arise in this age group and continue into the next decade result from consuming foods such as hamburgers, hot dogs, malts, and ice cream. All of these foods contain large amounts of animal fat and cholesterol and are low in polyunsaturated fats. It would be very difficult for a child growing up in the 1970's to avoid all of these. In fact, his unenlightened friends might well make him feel as though he were peculiar if he tended to avoid such all-American foods as we have listed above. So our job will be primarily to keep the total fat load as low as possible, granting that it will not be as low as we would like, but hoping that it will be considerably lower than children have been given in the past. If the child has been fed what basically is a low fat diet all his life, many of the high fat foods will actually be distasteful to him. When the youngster voluntarily selects low-fat foods in preference to those of high fat content, our program is a success.

The method of cooking is important. Fried foods are generally to be avoided. Meat should be cooked with no added fat and, in fact, can be cooked so that the fat within the meat melts and drains away. Teflon-lined cooking utensils have done away with the need for adding butter or other shortenings to the meat or vegetable. The use of ice milk rather than ice cream does lower the fat content moderately, but if you read the label you will see that there is still considerable butterfat present. My only suggestion is that the child be informed that ice cream and malts are food that he may have occasionally, but not something that he may have every day.

Bakery products present another problem in this age period. The labels of bakery products rarely give any idea of the amount of butterfat and egg yolk used. There is one very excellent bakery product on our low-fat diet list, angel food cake. This contains no shortening and no egg yolk, but does contain the protein portion of the egg as well as sugar and flour. Most children and adults like angel food cake, which has no cholesterol*. Another exception might be the diabetic, who should take the number of calories into consideration. In general, a low carbohydrate diet for long periods is unacceptable. There is a great deal of sound medical and nutritional information regarding reduced performance of work when carbohydrates are significantly restricted. Some current diet fads may be truly dangerous in this regard. Of course, we recognize that we all eat too much simple sugar, but the more complex carbohydrates and starches are necessary for proper functioning. I have told you in previous chapters that the child develops all of his

*The sugar and flour content may be a problem if the individual happens to have a carbohydrate-dependent type of hyperlipemia—high fat content of the blood.

fat cells by the time he is one year of age. This is almost true. There is another period in life when a few fat cells are formed. This is in the prepuberty period, sometime around the 10th to 12th year. This is especially noticeable in young girls; certainly, we do not wish to fat-starve them to the point where their figures might suffer in years to come. Actually, in this country it would be almost impossible to fat-starve anyone to that point; however, the point is made in order to remind you that over-feeding can produce additional fat cells that may be a problem later in life. Males apparently establish a few more fat cells at this time, but they do not become obvious until years later. The implication of our discussion is still moderation, especially moderation in the total number of calories consumed, with as much restriction as feasible in the level of fat consumption.

To summarize the ages 5 through 14, it is apparent that this is the safest period of life. The exciting process of growth and development continues. Intellectual stimulation and growth, physical stimulation and growth make a combination that is hard to beat. The warnings at this time are obviously motivated by concern over accidents. The development of safety habits and attitudes is paramount. At the same time, we want to avoid overfeeding and encourage reduction of fat intake. We are still looking to the future in the attempt to make the adult productive years healthful and safe. This is a decade of discipline; it is the responsibility of parents to see that good habits of eating and physical fitness are firmly instilled into the life style of the child.

IX. The Decade of Decision

Ages 15 Through 24

The lowest mortality existed in the decade that we have just completed, the 5-to-14 age group. The most rapid increase in the mortality rate occurs from the 15th to the 24th year. Note from Chart XIV that our death rate has jumped to 116.9 per 100,000 population. The death rate in the last decade was only 41.4 per 100,000; therefore, we have increased the death rate by 2.8 times as we move into this decade. No other decade represents such a significant increase in the death rate over the decade immediately preceding it. Only birth defects take fewer lives now than in the previous period. All other major entries show significant increases in the death rate. Infections and malignancy have modestly increased their death rates in this decade, while suicides have increased 23 times, and homicides have multiplied 13 times. This, in part, reflects the relatively small number of homicides and suicides in the 4-to-14 age group. The number is no longer insignificant. Accidents have increased 3.4 times. Major cardiorenal diseases have increased 3 times, and we are now listing for the first time complications of pregnancy, which represent 2 deaths per 100,000 in this age group.

The total population in the 15-to-24 age group in 1967

was 32,265,000. This number is modestly less than that one decade earlier. For rough calculations, if you wish to determine the exact number of patients dying in each category, multiply the number listed on the chart by 323, which will give you a reasonable approximation of the number of deaths in each category.

Accidents remain the largest killer in this age group. The 67.1 deaths per 100,000 from accidents alone is higher than deaths from all causes in the earlier decade. In terms of actual numbers, accidents took the lives of 21,645 in this teen-age and young adult group. Motor vehicle accidents took 15,646 lives in this category, easily leading all others as a cause of death. It is interesting to note that the total number of deaths in the 15-to-19 age group was slightly higher than in the 20-to-24 age group. This is evidence of developing stability as one reaches the mid-twenties. It is tragic that the young driver, the learner, is apparently cursed with more recklessness than ability. Males in this age group are killed approximately four times as often as females. Despite the rather extensive data in the accident mortality section of the *Vital Statistics* book, one occasionally has difficulty in grouping certain types of accidents together. For instance, it would seem that a large percentage of the motorcycle fatalities would occur in the age group we are now discussing. By going through the accident mortality tables, I came up with 1,971 motorcycle deaths. However, this is not broken down by age, and I have no way of knowing how many are in the 10-year period between ages 15 and 24. Compared to estimates of authors in the medical literature, this number would seem to be slightly low. Authors in the medical literature usually report the motorcycle mortalities per year as being somewhat above 2000. Perhaps 1967 was a better year than those referred to in other articles, or I must admit that the charts are ambiguous enough that I might lose a few motorcycle accidents in other categories. It has been recorded with reasonable accuracy that there were two million registered motorcycles in 1967. If one uses the round figure of 2000 deaths, this would mean that there are 100 deaths for every 100,000 registered motorcycles per year. Some improvement has occured since 1967. In 1971, 3,300,000 registered motorcycles resulted in 2410 deaths, or 72 deaths per 100,000 motorcycles per year. This is about double the death rate for registered automobiles. The high death rate that results from motorcycle crashes is apparently caused by the gross lack of protection to the body. When control of the vehicle is lost, the occupant is thrown to the ground with considerable velocity. A New York survey in 1968 indicated that in motorcycle accidents, 94.4 per cent of the time the occupants were significantly injured. The total number of 1967 deaths as approximately 2000 does not tell the entire accident story related to motorcycles. Precise figures again are hard to find, but it has been estimated that approximately 300,000 significant motorcycle injuries occurred in 1967. A survey made on the UCLA campus revealed that, although 55 per cent of the students at the University of California had automobile transportation and only 6.5 per cent used motorcycles, the number of students injured by motorcycles was greater than those injured by automobiles by a ratio of 2 to 1. The ratio of injuries to registered vehicles was therefore about 20 times greater for motorcycles than for cars. The so-called economy motor bike was actually an expensive form of transportation. Another author reports that, considering all types of injuries and the number of miles traveled, the motorcycle is 16 times as dangerous as the automobile and results in 5 times more deaths per mile on the highway. If we suffered the same death rate from automobiles that we have from motorcycles, the automobile death rate would be 250,000 each year.

As I see the many small motorcycles in our suburban area and our cities, I am first of all aghast to see that they rarely have leg guards; even my machine of 30 years ago had sturdy crash bars. I feel that there is an illusion of safety in small motorcycles. However, if the motorcycle is going at 20 miles an hour the human body becomes a missile with enough force to produce death. Smallness is certainly no guarantee of safety in motorcycles. The Committee on Medical Aspects of Automotive Safety has reported on motorcycle safety. The report appeared in *The Journal of the American Medical Association* in 1968.

This article lists all of the constructive things that can be done in operating a motorcycle. It, of course, recommends the protective headgear and eyeshields and emphasizes the fact that heavy clothing should be worn and that arms and legs should not be uncovered while riding. In addition, it lists many common-sense operational procedures such as not driving abreast, not driving on the shoulder or between traffic lanes, the avoidance of tailgating and, above all, driving in a defensive manner. All of these precautions apply to automobile safety, as well, but the motorcycle operator is so exposed, so unprotected, so vulnerable to flying gravel or the slightest miscalculation that all of these safety features become multiplied in their significance.

An extremely interesting article appeared in *The American Journal of Psychiatry* in 1970 by Dr. Armand Nicholi of the Harvard Medical School Psychiatry Department. He discusses the "Motorcycle Syndrome." The author presents an in-depth study of nine accident-prone motorcyclists and outlines their particular personality makeup. I am sure many motorcycle operators are stable citizens who wish to have an economical means of transportation. Yet, we are all aware of the image of the motorcyclist in the gang as portrayed by movies and television. Certainly, there does seem to be a personality type for which the motorcycle offers a tremendous ego crutch. The author describes the motorcycle as a powerful emotional prosthesis, an extension of what the rider conceives as masculine reassurance. The motorcycle helps him reassure himself that he is truly a man; apparently, this type of personality needs reassurance in this area. I frankly confess that I am not a psychiatrist and am often a little skeptical of what these analysts have to offer. However, the components of the motorcycle syndrome as listed by the previously mentioned author seem impressive:

1. Unusual preoccupation with the motorcycle.
2. A history of accident-proneness extending back to early childhood.
3. A persistent fear of bodily injury.
4. A distant conflict-ridden relationship with the father and a strong identification with the mother.
5. Extremely passive personality, with an inability to compete.
6. A defective self-image.
7. Poor impulse control.
8. Fear of, and counterphobic involvement with, aggressive girls.
9. Impotence and intense homosexual concerns.

Dr. Nicholi certainly does not wish to imply that all motorcycle operators fall into the above categories, but one must admit that there are some unusual traits that seem to be common to avid motorcycle fans.

Would I let my own son own a motorcycle? Certainly not—if I could help it. When a young man reaches adulthood and is self-supporting, I doubt that the parents can exert much influence. Certainly, I would strongly advise against its purchase, yet I would be forced to admit that I learned a great deal about the hazards of the road during my six-months' ownership of one in my youth. I would hope that, if my son did purchase a motorcycle, he would, like me, be more than happy to sell it in a short period of time.

In this decade between the 15th and the 24th year, 21,645 people were killed by motor vehicle accidents. That is a number we cannot ignore. We must examine it and investigate to learn if any substantial number of lives can be salvaged. We have already discussed the motorcycle, but this made up only 10 per cent of the deaths mentioned above. Regardless of the high accident rate on motorcycles, we must admit that, because of the tremendous number of automobiles, they involve the largest number of people. In diagnostic radiology we see many automobile accident victims. Those that are dead on arrival are not usually X rayed; only the critically or the painfully injured come for our services. I can think of nothing that would do more to make the young person in our age group interested in careful driving than to work in an emergency room or in a radiology department for a time. Business is always good on weekends and over long holidays. The pain and misery of accidents cannot be adequately described. Insurance companies can furnish a dollar figure. The department of labor statistics might give information on time missed from work, but there is no way anyone can impress upon you the misery and the pain of a severely traumatized human body. In preparing these sections on accidents, I am trying, not only to rely on my experience and prejudice, but to call on the medical literature, the legal literature, and some of the safety bulletins. It is also surprising how much information can be gleaned from newspapers, periodicals, and medical newspapers.

In automobile accidents it is the deceleration that kills. When an automobile moves forward at even a moderate rate of speed and strikes an immovable object, the body continues to move forward with significant force because of inertia. The type of trauma that results to the body depends on the point at which the deceleration impact is centered. We know from statistical data that approximately 60 per cent of automobile accident deaths result from injury to the head. Thirty per cent of the deaths follow primary injuries to the chest and abdomen; the other 10 per cent are caused by injuries to the extremities or are unclassified.

When the automobile stops suddenly, the body of the occupant tends to be thrown forward and upward. Since most modern cars, particularly the hardtop variety, have relatively little headroom, the head of the victim will be directed toward the top and front of the automobile. This is in the area of the sun visor. The head and face are literally smashed by the impact. This is a very common type of auto injury that arrives at our emergency rooms and X ray departments. These patients are sometimes blessed with unconsciousness. It can usually be determined in relatively short order that the chest and abdomen are essentially normal and that the only immediate risk to the victim's vital signs is aspirated saliva and blood. The airway is maintained, and the patient's head injury is assessed. Head injuries can be so severe that the patient cannot recover. However, early in the postaccident period it is difficult to separate this person from a patient who has signs of severe head injury because of edema and swelling. The latter patient will recover.

Therefore, patients are treated by support of their vital signs, and time separates the two groups for us. Another very disconcerting type of injury is the one that results in somewhat less brain damage, but in which the face is literally crushed. Fractures extend across the forehead and down through each side of the face bones. In examining this patient, if one places the index and third finger in the mouth and the thumb against the front teeth, it becomes apparent that the whole anterior face can be freely moved back and forth. After seeing such a case, you are not inclined to forget your seat belt and shoulder harness. Because of the large number of head and face injuries, I feel there is a place for some type of headgear in automobiles. Would crash helmets be too much? I am sure they would be ideal for protective purposes; however, knowing how difficult it has been to persuade people to use seat belts, I have little faith that they would accept crash helmets in autos. The "hard hat," the type worn by construction workers, might be more acceptable and should save many lives. To my knowledge, no one has recommended protective headgear for the automobile driver and passenger; however, it is so logical I feel it must be forthcoming.

Severe chest injuries, like severe head injuries, can be fatal immediately. The chest is suddenly stopped by the steering wheel, and the aorta is torn from the heart. This results in prompt death. Lesser degrees of chest trauma include penetration of the lung, tears with hemorrhage into the lung and, of course, the always painful multiple rib fractures. The collapsible steering column and again the shoulder and chest strap are extremely important.

Abdominal injuries can be painful and more subtle in their clinical manifestations. Tear of the liver, spleen, kidneys, or bladder can result in death by blood loss, infection, or irreparable damage to a vital organ. The intestinal tract may actually explode from the impact on the abdomen. This pours intestinal contents into the peritoneal space, and the next several weeks are spent recovering from the infection. I suggest that you never drive with a full bladder or a full colon. *Never drive after a large meal.* Overdistention of the intestinal tract or bladder predisposes to a traumatic rupture. It is a relatively easy and important safety measure to eat lightly and make frequent rest stops on automobile trips.

Some figures in regard to accidents and accident prevention seem to recur in all forms of literature. They are repeated so often that they become almost holy. Yet every now and then an article may come out, seemingly sincere statistically, that casts some doubt on the standard accepted data. For instance, a number of references state that half of our automobile fatalities involve the use of alcohol. Certainly, anyone who works around an emergency room or X ray department has the impression that, if anything, this is a low percentage. However, with such a statement we are probably reflecting our own prejudices. It is a fact that the alcoholic patient is such a repulsive, irritating person that we remember him more vividly than the sober accident victim. Nothing I can think of makes a greater impression on emergency room personnel and on people trying to take care of him than to have a belligerent, semiconscious patient who reeks with alcohol. For this reason I am sure that I and most medical personnel would estimate that at least half of the automobile accidents involve drunken drivers. It is also stated that at least half the deaths on the highway might be prevented by the use of seat belts; possibly 25 per cent could be avoided by the use of shoulder harnesses; and 7 per cent are caused by bad tires. Poor highway construction may cause another 10 per cent. All of this begins to make it appear that we have the means of preventing well over 100 per cent of all automobile deaths. I find it impossible to indulge in such optimism.

In general, there are three components in every accident. One is the highway, another is the automobile and its condition. The third and the most difficult to evaluate is the driver. These factors exist in a complex interrelationship. We will consider each of these separately, without attempting to oversimplify the problem.

My comments on the highway itself will be relatively short because it appears to have been studied the least. One or two points seem pertinent. It is significant that fatalities in relation to miles traveled are less than half on the multilane divided, limited-access highways, compared to those on the traditional parallel roadways. This super type of highway is more common in the United States than in other countries, but certainly is not limited to this country. The United States highway system carries double the traffic load of the European roadways, with a fatality rate in relation to miles traveled that is only half as great. This would imply that American highways are constructed with more inbuilt safety than the European roads. The next series of data is not quite so encouraging. On our interstate system, slightly over half of the fatal accidents occur off the road, and over 80 per cent of these off-the-road accidents involve fixed objects. This implies that more free space on each side of the roadway for the automobile to decelerate would be of value and that fixed objects should be kept at a minimum in this area. If you have traveled on European highways, you will recall that most of them offer little or no off-the-road deceleration space. The amount of land that can be consumed by highway construction is great, and the amount of land that is actually used depends on how precious that property is. In this country we have had extensive land and have been inclined to use it generously, at least when compared to roadways in other countries. However, the point is well made that a level deceleration space on each side of the road would be a very prominent safety feature, particularly if this safety area had a different type surface that would awaken the sleeping driver or arouse the semicomatose drunk. A certain number of fixed objects seem to be inevitable, but with some thought and consideration a certain number of these could be reduced, or break-away signs could be used. It would be ideal to put 50 or 100 yards of level deceleration space on each side of the two-lane road, but the land consumption of such an arrangement would be tremendous. If this land could be made productive as well as offer a safety barrier, the objection of land wastage could be reduced.

Volumes have been written concerning the role of the automobile in the prevention of accidental death. It seems that the greatest hope for improvement lies in better engineering. It is apparently easier to better the automobile than it is to improve the driver. Despite a great deal of driver education, the auto fatality rates remain relatively unchanged. Since 1967 there have been a number of improvements in autos that have not yet been completely evaluated. We might quote a number of sources however; the UCLA Trauma Research Group has offered some rather sensible points for consideration. They feel that improved window glass has reduced the number of severe face and head lacerations. They find the collapsible steering column and the padded instrument panel to be significant advances. All of these features make the cars made since 1967 safer than those manufactured before that time. They have also done studies in reference to car weight and deceleration and show without question that one is safer in a heavier car than in a light one. This should not come as a great surprise. It is sometimes referred to as the "tank syndrome"—there are obvious practical limitations. With the emphasis now on economy cars, safety research applicable to small automobiles is very important. Some Japanese work implies they can be made as safe as larger cars. Seat belts have undoubtedly given us the opportunity to reduce mortality, but these are dependent on use by the individual. Cars now manufactured have electronic devices to enforce the use of seat belts. The shoulder belt has been incompletely studied at this time; however, this UCLA Trauma Research Group reports instances in which they feel that the shoulder belt and lap belt combination has clearly resulted in the saving of life. Television reports regarding lap and shoulder belts state that to date there have been no fatal accidents to persons using lap and shoulder belts if the crash did not involve speeds of over 50 miles per hour. This is an extremely important observation and stresses how our lowered speed limits and safety straps could make real inroads on the magnitude of auto accident deaths. Side impact bars and headrests have become standard since 1969. The UCLA Group suggests that we drive only a car that weighs at least 3500 pounds and that has been manufactured since 1967. The lap belt and shoulder harness combination should be used by all adults, and the infant carrier shield system should be employed for children.

There is little doubt in my mind that Detroit will continue to improve the safety of its product. This is especially true if those of us who are interested in this feature continue to maintain pressure. At the present time the manufacturers are more involved in improving gas mileage and antipollution devices than safety factors. As these problems come under control, additional energy will be diverted to the safety of automobile construction. Newspapers and magazines have carried a number of reports concerning potential safety features. Air bags that inflate on contact have been widely discussed. Their efficiency is unproven, and some investigators seem skeptical. They are not effective at speeds greater than 50 miles per hour and despite their expense are no more effective than lap and shoulder straps at lower speeds. Their advantage, of course, lies in not requiring driver cooperation. Additional research needs to be done on a more resilient lining for the entire inner surface of the car. We might do well to talk to stock car race drivers and get their opinions of safety devices and automobiles. It is amazing how many crashes race drivers can have at high rates of speed and still survive. Obviously, a great deal of safety engineering has gone into their automobiles. Gene Murray of *The Kansas City Star*, interviewed a group of stock car drivers to acquire their impressions concerning automobile safety. They made many strong points, some of which are applicable to general motoring safety.

The drivers are securely strapped to the seats. All of the cars used in racing have reinforcing roll bars over the top and sides. If the car turns over, the top can support the entire weight, and the auto does not crush the driver. Several of the drivers interviewed commented on the impracticability of the popular hardtop automobiles; convertibles would fall in the same category. Racing drivers are also very much in favor of a special type of fuel container, the fuel cell, which prevents leakage of gasoline if a crash occurs. This, of course, would be more important to the stock car racer than to most of the general public. Their fuel is more volatile than the regular gas used by American drivers. Fire is a relatively uncommon complication of the usual traffic accident. Less than 2 per cent of automobile crash victims die of burns. Crash helmets have improved in design. Protective bumpers are now being produced. Additional support has been applied to the sides of current automobiles; however, to be truly effective, it needs to be increased and reinforced several fold. There is no question that there is plenty of room for improvement in the safety design of automobiles. I am optimistic that these improvements will come—they must!

Tires are an important and integral part of the automobile, yet most of us know very little about them except what we have learned from television and radio advertising. Such terms as "super premium" or "cat paws" give us very little in the way of real information in regard to tire quality. Some standard type of quality grading, whether set up by the government or by the industry, seems to be required. Once these standards are established, quality control would be easier, and hopefully fewer dangerous tires would appear on the highway.

The final and ultimate responsibility for automobile safety lies with the driver. It is true that the government has responsibility for providing safe roads. It is also true that the manufacturer has responsibility for making a safe automobile. Still, the ultimate responsibility for maneuvering his one- to three-ton missile about our streets and highways depends upon the man at the wheel. His physical condition is, of course, important, as is his mental attitude. His background and his training, especially in the area of accident prevention and control, are also vital factors. Man is a far more complex machine than the automobile or the highway. He can break down in a number of ways and in so doing be responsible for his death and that of others. The auto is rarely used as a device for deliberate homicide. However, as long as double indemnity life insurance is available, it will be a device for suicide. These suicides are hard to prove, but we all know they exist.

A number of features need to be considered when evaluating the driver's role in accidents The age of the driver is important. Drivers under 20 and over 70 have distinctly higher accident rates than those in the middle years.

An obvious and rather simple statement is that people who are sick should not drive cars. A diabetic who tends to faint from a lack of sugar or go into a coma when the sugar in the blood is too high is certainly a highway risk. Unless he is perfectly controlled, he should not drive. Persons who tend to faint for any reason are distinct highway hazards and, of course, there are those unanticipated illnesses such as heart attack or stroke that occasionally occur when the patient is driving. This happens all too often; the reasons for this will be discussed in our section on heart disease. Poor vision and poor hearing have been incriminated in auto accidents, and these physical handicaps should deny their victims the right to drive.

Alcohol and drugs reduce the driver's ability to respond and think and thus increase the probability of accidents. The extent of the risk depends upon the amount of alcohol consumed or the amount of alcohol in the blood at the time. As stated earlier, a frequently quoted figure in this country is that half of all vehicle accidents involve alcohol. The figures in the literature vary. A report from Baltimore covering the period 1951 to 1956 claimed 58.3 per cent. A report from the Mayo Clinic, in "Minnesota Medicine," in 1970 gave an estimated incidence of 46 per cent. The Grand Rapids Survey, which was one of the most carefully conducted studies on the role of drinking in accidents, attributed 21 per cent of accidents directly to alcohol. This study went into a great deal of detail and found that frequent, low-volume drinkers had fewer accidents than nondrinkers; however, it did confirm the fact that the extensive user of alcohol was the most serious offender. It has been stated by other groups that approximately half of all accidents involve alcohol and that half of these are problem drinkers rather than occasional drinkers. A relatively short editorial in *The Journal of Forensic Medicine* for October-December 1970 offers a worldwide evaluation of alcohol. It is of interest and considerable importance that alcoholism is virtually nonexistent in Israel. The number of persons arrested for drunkenness there is 0.74 for 10,000 population. A similar figure for England and Wales is 19 per 10,000. To my knowledge, no such figures are available for the United States. When blood levels of alcohol exceeding 50 mg per 100 cc were used in evaluating accidents in various countries, the United States figure was 58.3 per cent from Baltimore compared to 0.0 per cent for Israel, a country where alcoholism as a cause of auto accidents does not exist. The editor of the article to which I refer goes on to point out that Israel still has a significant number of accidents and, in fact, has more than many other countries. However as I look at the data presented, the death rate per 100,000 in Israel is 14. At the same time, in the United States, it is 26 per 100,000. This comes remarkably close to our magic 50 per cent figure quoted by so many people.

My prejudice may be showing, but it is consistent with that of many others. It seems to me that the role of alcohol in auto accidents is too great to be ignored. If 50 per cent of our fatal accidents involve significant amounts of alcohol, this should be the place where improvement can be achieved. Some may wish to rely on the wisdom of our courts and legislators to find the best corrective methods. I have another suggestion that may sound vaguely familiar: "If you drive, don't drink."

Another promising approach involves a device that General Motors is developing and is called Phystester, which most of us have seen on television. This requires the driver to remember a series of five digits and punch them on the keyboard in the proper sequence before his car will start. Various modifications can be added to this to make it slightly more complex, and this should have some potential in keeping the drunk driver from starting his car. However, I would not purchase one on my car because I don't need it. I am sure that the chronic alcoholic would not purchase one because it would ground him in unfavorable situations. Therefore the device, if it is found acceptable, must be made mandatory on all automobiles, and this will most certainly increase the cost of the auto. After some experience with the device, it might lower insurance rates enough to pay for itself. It is more likely to be abandoned.

Complications of Pregnancy, Abortion, and Childbirth

As one reviews the general statistics in the area of pregnancy complications, childbirth, and abortion, one finds that 7 deaths occurred between the ages of 10 and 14 and that no deaths are listed after the age of 50. There was a total of 987 deaths in the year 1967 in all age groups of women as complications of pregnancy, childbirth, or the immediate post-delivery period. In the decade of the 15-to-

24 age group, there were 347 deaths. The death rate per 100,000 is higher in this category than for any other decade, principally because of the high mortality rate in the young pregnant patient. The highest single cause of death in this group is listed as toxemia of pregnancy.

It was in 1968 that legislation to liberalize abortion was introduced and then discussed by two groups—the pro- and the anti-abortionists. These arguments continue. One of the arguments presented by physicians' groups in favor of liberalizing abortion was the desire to remove the patient from the hands of the criminal abortionist who "had a very high mortality and morbidity rate" and to bring the woman who was determined to have an abortion into the protected environment of a fine hospital and well-trained personnel. To those of us who had witnessed the death of young girls through sepsis following abortion, this sounded like a very logical argument. I doubt if anyone checked the statistics to challenge that contention. In 1967 abortion by all means, criminal and therapeutic, took a total of 160 lives. I do not wish to enter the abortion argument. I mentioned earlier that there may be social reasons for abortion, but if you believe that abortion is the taking of one life to prevent another from becoming a mortality statistic, the numbers balance out rather poorly. Approximately 30,000 legal abortions are performed each month. To balance that number against the 160 maternal deaths that occurred in 1967 would seem to weight the scales a bit to one side.

Maternal mortality statistics seem to be quite good. Nine hundred and eighty-seven deaths occurring during delivery of 3,520,959 infants would seem to be an acceptable mortality rate. Of course, we should not be satisfied with this. I hope the rate can be improved by both preventive measures and medical treatment. In terms of numbers, more success can be found in reducing premature births than in lowering maternal mortality. It is logical to assume that both statistics will improve together.

Malignant Diseases—Ages 15-24 and 5-14

Certain similarities in the types of malignancy occur in the two decades between ages 5 and 24. There are also some apparent differences; for this reason I have elected to discuss the two together. Most of us think of the malignancies that involve late childhood, adolescence, and young adulthood as being similar in type. As a general rule, this is true. However, when one tries to make that assumption for as long a period of time as 20 years, certain inconsistencies can be expected. When thinking of malignancies in young adults, most of us in diagnostic radiology think of brain tumors, leukemias, bone tumors, and lymphomas. Lymphomas, as you will recall, are malignancies that arise from lymph nodes. Bone tumors below the age of five are rare. These four areas produce most of the malignancies in the age groups to which we are referring. The following chart will both support this statement and also emphasize its inconsistencies:

	Ages 5-14	Ages 15-24
Brain	538	294
Bone	188	248
Leukemia	1279	675
Lymphoma	323	596
All other areas	383	1019
Total	2711	2832

The first noticeable similarity is the fact that the total number of deaths from malignancy in the two age groups is virtually the same. However, remember that the age group 5 through 14 embraces the largest number of people of any decade in 1967. This shows the value of using death rate statistics rather than actual numbers; there has been a definite increase in the death rate for malignancy in the 15-to-24 age group compared to the younger decade. As one looks across the chart, it is apparent that brain tumors and leukemia are decreasing. An even more striking difference in the two age categories relates to the entry, "all other areas." The four types of tumors listed account for 86 per cent of the malignancies in the 5-to-14 age group, but the same four areas account for only 64 per cent in the 15-to-24 age group.

This large number of malignant tumors that fall outside of the usual group intrigued me enough to go back to the vital statistics detail section to see if there was any particular area that deserved additional listing. I was surprised to find that in the 15-to-24 age group at least one person died of every known malignancy that is classified by the vital statistics department, with the exception of malignancy of the lip and malignancy of the larynx. In other words, by the time the person reaches the twenties he is subject to every known malignancy. Cancer of the lip is certainly an understandable exception, since there were a total of only 143 deaths from this entity at all ages. This is a very slow-growing tumor and is usually treated very adequately. The absence of involvement of the larynx with malignant disease in our young age group is not explained quite so easily; however, the mortality detail statistics indicate that no one died of cancer of the larynx until the 30-34 year age group was reached. All other organs were subject to malignant disease in the 15-to-24 category. I was interested to note that there were 42 primary carcinomas of the respiratory tract; 27 were in males and 15 in females. Cancer of the breast took the life of 22 females in this age group; coincidentally, cancer of the cervix took exactly the same number, 22 in 1967. Cancer of the ovary was a surprise. Here 83 girls died of this form of malignancy.

We are a long way from preventing deaths in this age group from malignancy. Our only hope in lowering the death rate is to do a better job medically. We like to think that earlier diagnosis can improve survival rates. This is true in some instances of bone tumor and possibly even an occasional brain tumor. There are also types of leukemias and lymphomas that, when treated aggressively during the early stages, seem to enjoy longer survival rates. Hodgkins' disease, a special type of lymphoma, certainly falls in this category. Dr. Henry Kaplan of Stanford has stimulated many radiotherapists in the country to aggressively irradiate Hodgkins' disease, and this seems to improve the survival statistics. Drug therapy with leukemia has prolonged life but, as we mentioned earlier, it is difficult to speak in terms of cure when discussing leukemia. Of the many other tumors that occur in the 15-to-24-year-old group, a number of cures are obtained. However, the cure rate is much lower than I like to admit. I cannot give you accurate overall statistics but, as a general rule, the survival rates tend to be poorer for the young patient (5-24) than for the middle-aged and elderly patients. It is also less encouraging than in the very young (28 days to 4 years).

In matters of disease and health there seems to be an unreasonable amount of luck, or the lack of it, in life. It is as though all of the diseases and all of the catastrophes and all of the minor things that happen to people are listed on separate slips of paper and put into a large bag. Then each year each one of us is asked to reach down into the bag and select one. Those who are lucky may get acne or a broken bone, a laceration, or possibly be given another year's reprieve. But somewhere in that bag there is a brain tumor, leukemia, and so forth. And since the bag must be emptied according to the rules of statistics each year, there are bound to be some who draw the bad options. As we discuss the next few decades, I will point out ways in which we can improve our chances in life, but unfortunately we can never improve to the point of perfection, and every so often one of those miserable disastrous diseases is going to be drawn by you, your family, or your friends.

Suicide

Suicide ranks as the fourth leading killer in the age group 15 to 24. Its 23-fold increase over the previous decade represents the largest increase on our chart. As we go through subsequent decades, we will find that the incidence of suicide increases each decade until we reach age 65. In 1967 we recorded no suicides in the 5-to-9 age group. There were 121 in the 10-to-14 age group. In the decade from 15 to 24, 2244 deaths are classified as suicides. Our vital statistics book gives us very little other detail about suicide. It does tell us that most suicides are carried out by means of firearms and that suicide by poisoning is the next most common method.

Other sources give additional data on this entity. It has been reported that among college students suicide is now the second leading cause of death. The rate is 50 per cent higher among students in college than among noncollege Americans of comparable age. It tends to be even higher in Britain than in the United States. The British report 19.3 deaths per 100,000 from suicides, while the American college student has a suicide rate of 10.5 per 100,000. Both of these figures are above the overall rate of 7.0 per 100,000 listed in our chart.

In more mature persons, suicide generally occurs for one of two reasons. The person is realistically in a hopeless situation, perhaps with an incurable malignancy and suicide is a relatively logical solution. This is a way out that will involve less pain and less trouble and expense for his family. If I may use the term, this would seem to be a logical suicide. However, these are relatively small in number. A far greater number of suicides result from mental depressions. This is simply one of the forms of mental illness in which patients cannot put their problems in proper perspective and find themselves becoming more and more depressed. Suicide becomes an end forced on the person by his illness. There is some question whether adolescent suicides are related to either of these two mechanisms. One author will say that depressions are virtually unheard of in adolescents and young adults, while the next author contends that depressions exist in adolescents and young adults, but that they take a different form and are much more difficult to recognize than in adults. Not being involved in the psychiatric field, I feel no inclination to explain the differences of opinion. The important aspect from our standpoint is that all authors maintain that a very high percentage of suicides is preventable. The one exception might be the suicide of logic. Certainly, in mature adults, if the depression can be identified and treated, the tendency toward suicide, and therefore suicide itself, disappears. If depression does not occur in the adolescent or young adult or if it is so difficult to identify that some experts claim that it does not occur, we need to look for other signs and symptoms to warn us of impending disaster.

In the adolescent, more important contributing factors to suicide would include acting out of angry feelings, attempt at manipulation of the environment, and the feeling of being cornered. In the child, manipulative behavior such as that required for punishing parents and impulsive verbal acts are often causally related to suicide statements and threats. Certainly, many parents have been told by the disgruntled child, "You will miss me when I am gone" or something of this type. This is also related to the fact that children, adolescents, and even some young adults have not established in their minds the fact that death is an irreversible act. They tend to feel that they can commit the act of suicide, observe the sorrow of the parents at the funeral, then come back, and everyone will be forgiven, and life will continue as before. This lack of a fixed death concept probably contributes to suicide in the adolescent period.

Not all suicides exhibit such infantile logic. Some involve romantic problems, pregnancy, or fear of punishment by parents or society because of pregnancy or social problems. This fear of social punishment becomes so great that life does not seem worthwhile. In one series of girls 17 and 18 years of age, 30 per cent were married, separated, widowed, unwed mothers, or unwed and pregnant. In boys homosexuality was frequently reported. Either the boy was active homosexually or feared that he was not normally heterosexual.

The role of suicide in the college student is somewhat different from those listed above, although many motives are similar. Causes that seem more pertinent in the college group include problems of identity, academic competition, financial pressure, drugs, and even the place of one's residence. Students who received educational grants that are dependent on maintaining a certain academic level are under tremendous pressure, and this has been known to be a source of suicide in a very intellectual group of students. Probably the most important cause in the student group was difficulty in establishing one's identity. The most frequent single comment made about this group of suicide victims by their colleagues has been that no one really seemed to know the victim. This is especially a factor in the freshman who arrives on the college campus after having been a success in his local high school. In college he finds considerably more competition and realizes that he is not an outstanding individual, but one of many people who compose a homogeneous group. In such a situation our student may well feel loss of identity. He will experience a sense of loss because of his separation from family and friends.

If life is to be meaningful to any of us, we must be able to work with other people but, above all, we must occupy a position that we, as individuals, feel is important. Our position, whether it be social or professional, must be such that no one else can fill that role. This is the real meaning of identity. When one tends to lose his identity or his self-esteem at any age, the chances of suicide mount considerably. However, in the adolescent or particularly the student group, this becomes a very important factor.

Let me sum up some of the ways in which authors suggest that the presuicide victim may be identified. Suicide threats may or may not be a serious sign; it depends entirely upon how the threat is expressed. A casual remark such as, "I think I will kill myself" probably has little or no meaning. However, if such a remark is directed to a parent or sibling or to a professional person when there is little or no emotional context, the threat becomes considerably more serious. Suicide intent may be expressed in more indirect ways, such as changes in behavior, withdrawal from friends, a drop in school performance, or a general change of mood. When these are accompanied with some of the predisposing pressures that we have listed earlier, they should be taken as very serious signs. In the younger child, even as early as ages 6 through 12, self-administered poisoning, even though the attempt was not even partially successful, should be construed as a serious emotional disturbance. Some authors feel that accidental poisonings after the age of 7 are the exception rather than the rule and that our poison centers might well serve as a key point in the identification of the potential suicide child. In older persons, particularly college students or adolescents, the person committing suicide had confided his intentions to at least one other person. A significant number of people committing suicide leave suicide notes, many of which are written some time prior to the actual act. When the adolescent shows a change in behavior, particularly if he becomes withdrawn, seldom leaves his room, tends to eat poorly, and his ability to concentrate reaches a low level, it is time for someone to identify this youngster and get him to a physician.

There were 21,325 suicides in all age groups in 1967. Deaths to the number of 2244 in the age group 15 to 24 in one year are too many. The number may actually have been higher, for some of the accidents may have been suicides. This is a very preventable cause of death. Certainly, the suicide prevention rate far exceeds our cure rate for malignancy. The situation requires observation and activity on the part of the potential victim's friends and relatives. The victim may seek help on his own, but this is not the general rule. He truly "needs a little help from his friends."

Looking Ahead from a Decade of Decision

The years prior to the age of 15 may well be classified as the years of discipline. It is in these early years that training is accomplished, respect is achieved, and the child is given a solid foundation on which he can make decisions. By the time the youngster has reached the age of 15 and certainly by the time he is involved in the decade between 15 and 24, he must make certain decisions. It is because of this shift in responsibility that we suggested that diet training, accident prevention and physical training start very early in life. Those of us who are interested in preventive medicine must suggest remedies ahead of realities. We have been advocating the low-fat, low-cholesterol, moderate-caloric-intake type of diet. We have told you this may be helpful in preventing heart disease in later years.

In each of the sections in which we look ahead, we must ask you to accept the fact that there are some things that should be avoided. We will develop the details as the pertinent decade arrives. Needless to say, in thinking primarily of prevention, one may deal with current decisions and current attitudes. This is particularly true when speaking in terms of accidents. On the other hand, it may be necessary to make decisions now that will pay off only after several decades. With this preface, we approach our future planning with the same attitude we have used in the past chapters.

We assume that the disciplines that we have suggested for diet in the earlier years have now become established routine. If this is true, you are normal in weight for your height. However, by the time one reaches the end of this decade a complication arises. Most people marry by the time they reach the mid-twenties. The habits of two people must then be merged into a single new household. Differences in eating habits are only one of many changes in life style that must be resolved. As a general rule, it is the female member of the couple who prepares the food and establishes most of the eating habits. Fortunately, there has been considerable publicity suggesting that the care and feeding of husbands should be not only pleasant, but healthful. So most brides are receptive to suggestions that will result in a longer and more healthful life for her, her husband, and her future family. The suggestions we have made in previous chapters might well constitute an early marital agreement. Milk means skim milk. Yellow spread for bread means corn oil margarine; cheaper margarines usually are lard-based and offer no improvement over butter. It would be best if there were no skillet in the house. Eggs, preferably without yolks, or egg substitutes are used for cooking, and desserts for the most part are fresh fruit. Here we are emphasizing the fact that this decade is a time for making decisions. No one will ridicule you if you continue the same sloppy scrambled eggs, ice cream, and greasy tid-bit existence of most Americans. However, this is a time in life in which you can make fundamental decisions that may truly increase the life span of all members of your family.

It is appropriate to state that those populations that live longest and apparently best are those that follow our rules. In the May 1973 *Reader's Digest,* Dr. Alexander Leaf summarizes his *National Geographic* report and reviews the findings of others as they study those areas where life to age 100 is commonplace. The dietary findings have an obvious common factor—total calories are moderately reduced, but the calories derived from fat, especially animal fat (high in cholesterol and saturated fatty acids), are markedly reduced. In some instances the fat calories ingested are only one-fourth the fat consumed by the average American.

The same preventive measures include an exercise program. Instead of curling up on the divan after dinner before the television, take a stroll through the park or a bicycle ride, which will not only be more pleasant, but infinitely healthier. Since we would like to see the male member of this marriage become more vigorous, some additional program may be needed for him. Some physical activity outside of the house is a very constructive act for both members of the family.

Other decisions concerning your social activities and health will be made in part if not in total during this decade. What role is alcohol going to play in your lives as individuals and as a couple over the next 50 years? Here again is a decision only you can make. You can find plenty of advice in regard to making this decision. In most instances this advice will be more emotional than scientific. In fact, you can get almost any advice you like, depending upon the source. The WCTU will certainly give you one type of advice, while the winetasters' guild or *Playboy* magazine may give you an entirely different idea. I will here try to relate only a few ideas, which we will discuss further in subsequent chapters. Even recently, it was felt that alcohol had considerable beneficial physiological effects. When I was in medical school we were led to believe that arteriosclerosis could in part be prevented by judicious use of alcohol. No one in his right mind has ever advocated alcoholic excess. It was also felt that alcohol had a number of psychological benefits; even to this day we cannot in all honesty deny this claim. The problem of alcoholic excess is one that is familiar to everyone. Alcohol is an addicting drug.

Only in the last six or seven years have articles appeared in the medical literature suggesting that even the predinner cocktail, if used regularly, might have some long-range deleterious effect. We have already described the problems related to automobile accidents. We know that liver damage can occur even with moderate long-term usage of alcohol, and these facts must be weighed against the psychological benefits of the drug. The psychological benefits that occur are dependent entirely upon the individual and his need for a psychological crutch. We will evolve more medical facts as our consideration of the decades advances.

There are definite medical contraindications against alcohol in any form, and these can best be described by your individual physician. In general, they apply to any form of liver disease and some forms of heart disease. I intend to demonstrate that the medical attitude toward alcohol has tended to swing from one of moderate support to one of restrained opposition. As evidence mounts, attitudes may change further. At the moment, alcohol is regarded more and more critically by physicians.

If alcohol does offer some physiological risk, one might reasonably ask if there are some drugs that can furnish a psychological lift and still not produce physiological damage. We honestly have no good answers to this question. Alcohol has been consumed in one form or another as far back as there is recorded history, and we still have some reservations about its effect in various areas. Marijuana, which to my knowledge would be the only reasonable challenger to alcohol, has had far too few clinical trials and too few years of observation to clarify its effect. Certainly, a compound that is entirely safe to the human mind and body and that would give a psychological lift to a person would be a very valuable adjunct to life. To my knowledge, no such drug exists. Drugs are prescribed for particular reasons and therefore must always be of sufficient therapeutic value to warrant any side effects the drug may exert. If we rely on some of the reports on marijuana, it may be that this is the ideal drug that can give mankind tremendous emotional and psychological satisfaction. However, not all reports are this glowing. In the October 2, 1972 issue of *The Journal of the American Medical Association,* Drs. Harold Kulansky and W. T. Moore of the University of Pennsylvania report on "Effects of Chronic Marijuana Usage." They report evidence to indicate that marijuana may produce permanent damage to the cerebral cortex. My reaction is one of interest. Psychological effects of the chronic type are also described; if this is associated with permanent brain damage, as the University of Pennsylvania group suggests, the price of this psychostimulator is too high. Male impotence has been reported as a complication of marijuana. Those who experiment with this compound must accept the fact that they are running a risk of unknown degree. In light of current evidence, I will do everything possible to discourage anyone near and dear to me from participating in such experiments. My feeling is that some lung or liver damage from this compound will result from long-term usage.

One other decision regarding a matter of health may well be made in this decade. This involves the use of tobacco. Here, from a medical standpoint, there need be no hedging. The medical literature is replete with reports on the effects of tobacco, particularly cigarettes. The evidence against this habit and its role in health is so overwhelming that one cannot help but wonder why the Federal government has not totally outlawed tobacco. Most radiologists and physicians dealing with chest diseases were against tobacco long before the Surgeon General issued his first report in 1964. It is virtually impossible to think of anything that is new and bad that has not already been said about tobacco. Whenever opinion becomes so lopsided, one wonders whether there is room for a contrary opinion. Shortly after the Surgeon General's strong statement, I admit that I wondered whether I might not have been wrong in my very early critical attitude toward cigarettes. Search as I may for something in their favor, I can find nothing to encourage the use of tobacco. I may, however, have found an explanation for the government's failure to act against tobacco. One need not have a very long memory to recall that cyclamates were taken from the market with only a fraction of the evidence against them that exists against tobacco. There may well be two reasons for not taking cigarettes off the market. We have already suggested that we have a population problem, and in terms of population control the government certainly must move very carefully and discreetly. The continued use of cigarettes, particularly in large quantities, offers at least a partial solution to this problem. The American Cancer Society reports, and we have no reason to think that this is an exaggeration, that average life expectancy is reduced by approximately six years in smokers. (See Appendix, Chart XXXI.) This is especially true of those who start smoking in the decade with which we are dealing. A little arithmetic gives you some striking dollar and cents figures. We know, for instance, that in 1967 there were approximately 19 million people over the age of 65. We also know that approximately 40 per cent of the population smokes; 40 per cent of 19 million people is 7,600,000. We know also that the average Social Security payment and benefits is approaching $3000 per year. Therefore, in any given year 7,600,000 people would receive $22,800,000,000 in Social Security benefits. If we then multiply that number by the six years of reduced life expectancy, we have a total of $136,800,000,000 saved. That is a significant amount of money Uncle Sam saves while simultaneously accomplishing a degree of population control without ever passing one bit of unpopular legislation!

I am being facetious, of course, in my previous remarks. I do not seriously believe that our government is a vindictive one. However, in any situation in which it is economically unfavorable for people to live for a long period of time, I doubt that they can expect much support or encouragement, or even good advice, from those people or that government that stands to lose by that longevity. Therefore, you best get your health advice, especially in terms of death prevention, from someone who does not stand to lose from your success.

The interrelationship of the Surgeon General's report, the tobacco lobby, and Congress is an intriguing one. No one person can possibly know the whole story of how so little happened after such an important report on a situation dangerous to the public health was so publicized. While there must have been some public apathy, Congress surely listened to interests of pressure groups rather than scientists. Susan Wagner tells the story in a journalistic, unbiased way in her book, *Cigarette Country*.

It is especially important that the use of tobacco not be started early in life. The effects of tobacco are cumulative. We speak of tobacco exposure in terms of pack years. One pack year means a pack per day for a year. Two pack years means two packs a day for one year or one pack a day for two years. Thus, we can quantitate tobacco usage quite satisafactorily. We do not have as good a method for quantitating alcohol usage, although amount drunk per average day is an acceptable figure. When cigarette usage is started early in life, it is easy to see how a large number of pack years can be acquired at a relatively young age. There is no "safe number of pack years." Since the effects are cumulative, the more pack years, the more danger there is. Anyone who has acquired 20 pack years of exposure has certainly placed himself in a dangerous range. If one started smoking at age 15, it is easy to see how the 20 pack years might well be acquired under the age of 40.

The concept of pack years will be applied in subsequent discussions. At this moment we are advising you categorically to stop the use of cigarettes. You can never have fewer pack years than you have right now. If you have not started the use of tobacco, I can assure you there is no health advantage to the use of this substance. I can also assure you that it plays a very dominant role in the early death of a number of our citizens. If you can think of better reasons to smoke than the ones I can offer against the use of tobacco, then proceed with its use, but remember that you have been advised. It is your decision. Once again we remind you that the decade from age 15 to 24 is the decade of decision.

X. The Decade of Duty
Ages 25 Through 34

Mental and physical growth and development, physical maturation, and increasing responsibility do not come in a stepwise fashion with decade divisions as we are presenting them here, but rather as a smooth ascending line until the peak is reached. It is also certain that the diseases to which each decade is subject are not specifically isolated to that decade, but tend to blend with other decades as a function of time. Certain diseases reach their peak incidence early in life and then decrease. Other diseases tend to start at a relatively low incidence and then progressively increase. Comparing the decade from 25 to 34 with the previous decade, you will see that certain causes of death have peaked out and that others are showing rather striking increases.

Chart XV lists the leading causes of death in persons between the ages of 25 and 34. Like the previous charts, it has been derived from the 1967 *Vital Statistics of the United States*.

In 1967, the total population of this age group was 22,818,000. This means that, if you wish to derive the actual numbers of death for a given entry in the chart, you may multiply the mortality rate figure by 228. The resulting figure, while slightly low, will be reasonably close. It is clear that the leading cause of death is unchanged from that in the previous decade. It is still accidents. The rate is 52 per 100,000, which is definitely less than in the preceding decade. This will be the last decade in which accidents will be the leading cause of death. Of course, accidents will continue to be fatal in every decade, but the peak incidence of accidents as a cause of death occurred in the 15-to-24-year age group with a rate of 67.1 per 100,000. As people become more mature and accept more responsibility, they also show more caution. Alternatively, one may say that the person who has been able to survive the hectic years of the teens and the early twenties is by nature a more cautious person. Although motor vehicle accidents remain the primary killer, at this time it seems to be inappropriate to discuss accidents further, even though this is the area that takes the largest number of lives for the given decade.

Infections as a cause of death show only a modest increase from the earlier decade. The number of deaths from pneumonia is almost identical to that seen in the earlier decade. The total number of deaths from infectious hepatitis is slightly less; however, the death rate is approximately the same.

The incidence of malignancy has slightly more than doubled from the previous decade; however, deaths from leukemia, brain tumors, and bone tumors continue to decrease, while most of the increase in tumor deaths occurs as the result of malignancies arising in other organ systems. The lymphomas are continuing to increase, although at a slightly slower rate than was seen over the past two decades.

Homicides and suicides have both increased by a factor of two over the previous decade. Suicides tend to increase each decade. Mental and reactive depressions become the primary cause of suicide from the early thirties through the later years. These mental illnesses carry a very promising cure rate when actively treated by the physician.

Homicides, on the other hand, are generally acts of passion or anger. Our official statistics list 3281 people as victims of homicide between the ages of 25 and 34 in 1967. Of these, 79 per cent were male, 21 percent were female. Seventy per cent of all homicides were carried out by means of firearms or explosives. The incidence of homicide in this country is generally higher than that in older European societies. Some psychiatrists feel that our highly individualistic heritage makes it difficult for people to live in crowded circumstances. There is certainly no way in which such opinions can be quantitated and scientifically evaluated. My personal impression, equally difficult to prove, is that the availability of guns in this country is in part to blame. A disagreement between Europeans may end as a fist fight or a make-believe duel, whereas in the United States the same argument ends in a murder when a gun is so readily available. From my standpoint, a way of reducing the number of homicides would be to limit or eliminate the availability of guns. This is obviously a superficial therapeutic solution. A more basic approach would be to eliminate the underlying anger and conflict that fueled the original argument. Human nature being what it is, I am rather pessimistic of success on this basis. However, I have pointed out in the previous discussion on growth and development that we have hopefully created in the infant and child an understanding of safety and consideration for others, and that, through sports and interpersonal relationships, we have helped him to develop an attitude of healthful respect for his associates.

Complications of pregnancy, abortion, and childbirth are decreased from the previous decade. This is primarily because of the elimination of the very young from the pregnant population and some decrease in the number of deliveries. Major cardiovascular and renal disease is showing a steady increase in mortality figures. The present decade rate of death is 22.3 per 100,000, which is approximately three times that of the previous decade. This threefold increase is one that we must accept, for it will continue. We shall discuss this category in some detail, but this discussion will be deferred until the role of this disease as a massive killer becomes more manifest.

Cirrhosis of the Liver

In 1958, the death rate per 100,000 from cirrhosis of the liver was 10.8. Every year since that time there has been an increase in the number of deaths from this disease. In 1967, the death rate reached 14.1. This represents nearly a 40 per cent increase in the death rate in the last ten years. Our 1971 data indicate that cirrhosis kills 15.5 persons per 100,000. Of all the other diseases to which man is heir, only cancer of the lung and pulmonary emphysema have subjected the public of the United States to such a disastrous increase in mortality in the last ten years. (See Appendix, Chart XXVIII.)

Before discussing cirrhosis of the liver, it is appropriate to make a few general but basic comments in reference to the organ, its functions, and its role in our basic life processes. The liver is a relatively large wedge-shaped organ in the right upper abdomen. It is directly beneath the right diaphragm, and in normal-sized adults it weighs approximately four pounds. Because of its unique functions, it has an equally unique blood supply. Arterial blood is carried to the liver by means of the hepatic artery, but this supplies only 25 per cent of the total blood flow to the organ. The remainder of the blood supply to the liver comes as venous drainage from the gastrointestinal tract. This venous supply of blood to an organ is unique. This enables food or poisons absorbed from the gastrointestinal tract to pass through the liver before they enter the general systemic circulation. The liver is not a physically active organ such as the heart, but is a tremendously active chemical factory. The research chemist and the biochemist have a heyday when they meet to talk about or investigate the liver functions. Many different compounds are brought to the liver. Some are simple sugars, others are relatively complex carbohydrates and starches; others are proteins with molecules of various sizes and fats of varying types, all of which must be broken down and stored or possibly resynthesized before being returned to the blood as usable fuel for the rest of the body. It is not surprising that numbers of bacteria and viruses are also absorbed from the intestinal tract and that these come to the liver, which serves as our first line of defense. The liver also plays a vital role in the circulation of the bile, which is formed of breakdown-products of the red blood cells and bile salts. These are taken to the liver and again run through the chemical factory and excreted into the gastrointestinal tract in the form of bile. If obstruction by means of stones or tumor occurs between the liver and the intestinal tract, patients become jaundiced. Jaundice can also occur when the liver itself becomes affected and cannot carry out its function of transporting the red-cell breakdown products into the gastrointestinal tract.

Over the last ten years, many practitioners of radiology and nuclear medicine have become extremely interested in organ imaging. This technique is carried out by giving the patient a radioactive compound, which goes to a specific organ; a radiation detection device makes it possible to map and outline the position of the radioactive material. Thus, it is possible to obtain a specific image of a given organ without interference from other body structures in the area. This specialty has come of age only in the last decade. I mention this only because of some of our experience in dealing with organ-imaging chemicals. It was very easy to find a compound that was concentrated by the liver; many different radioactive compounds can be used for imaging the liver with isotope techniques. However, the real problem was finding chemicals that went to other organs and not to the liver. Imaging the pancreas has been extremely difficult because it is close to the liver anatomically and because virtually every compound that goes to the pancreas is taken up with almost equal or even greater avidity by the liver. One of my colleagues remarked that we would probably never adequately visualize organs in the area of the liver simply because the liver itself was such an efficient garbage disposal unit that virtually every chemical injected or taken orally was concentrated there to a high degree, making it difficult to achieve visualization of neighboring structures. These comments are made only to emphasize the role of the liver in terms of food metabolism, drug utilization, detoxification, and all forms of chemical activity. The heart may be the mechanical pump of the body, the urinary tract is the plumbing system, the brain is the site of thought and neuromuscular control, but the liver is the chemical factory and source of fuel for all the other structures.

Philosophers and thinkers are certain that the soul resides in the brain. Poets and romanticists are certain that the soul resides in the heart. But the chemist and many physicians are equally certain that the soul must reside in the liver.

Medical historians attribute the first description of cirrhosis of the liver to Laënnec, a French physician who practiced in the early 1800's. He coined the word cirrhosis from the Greek *kirrhos* meaning "of yellow colour." Despite our association of Laënnec with cirrhosis of the liver, Dr. Charles Davidson, in his book on liver abnormalities, states that actually the first descriptions of this disease should be attributed to William Harvey, whose principal fame rests on the discovery of blood circulation. The importance of the color that Laënnec emphasized has been for the most part forgotten, and cirrhosis to most physicians now means sclerosis (an English word), or scarring and hardening. It is true that the liver of a patient suffering from this disease is yellow in color, but it is classically hard and knobby. It is contracted in size and is very fibrotic and stiff.

Other diseases such as chronic obstruction of the bile duct and chronic infection result in liver damage and produce cirrhosis. However, the most common cause of cirrhosis is chronic alcoholism. We should clarify one point: When speaking of cirrhosis of the liver, we are not specifically speaking of alcoholism, but of a disease process that involves the liver. Not all alcoholics develop cirrhosis of the liver; it is estimated that only between 10 and 30 per cent of alcoholics develop the disease. The converse is also true: Not all cirrhosis of the liver is caused by alcoholism. It is difficult to obtain good statistics to evaluate the percentage of cirrhosis of the liver caused by alcoholism, but the best data seem to imply that approximately three-fourths of all cases of cirrhosis may be attributed thereto. Those cases of cirrhosis not alcoholic in origin are referred to as cryptogenic. They are usually thought to be the end result of chronic hepatitis or caused by abnormal metabolites stored in the liver. The frightening increase in the death rate from cirrhosis of the liver is presumably related to the increased alcohol consumption throughout the country. In 1967, there were 27,816 deaths from cirrhosis of the liver; however, only 918 occurred in the decade between the ages of 25 and 34. The peak death rate incidence occurs at approximately age 50 and falls rather strikingly in later years, implying that this is one disease that is inconsistent with longevity.

From this brief description of the physiology of the liver, one can with some imagination, grasp the various manifestations of this disease. Certainly, metabolism will be less efficient than in the normal state, and this reflects itself in a general cachexia or wasting appearance of the patient. Even more striking are the circulatory changes brought about by the high resistance of the scarred liver as it serves as a dam to the strong flow of blood from the gastrointestinal tract. This damming effect results in the weeping of some of the plasma into the abdominal space. Because of the increased pressure within the vessels, collateral roots are established, and the blood returns to the systematic circulation from the intestinal tract, bypassing the liver. The picture of the patient with cirrhosis is now becoming more complete. In addition to the malnourished appearance of the extremities, the abdomen protrudes and is filled with fluid, and many dilated vessels appear on its surface. Other reflections of this collateral venous return involve hemorrhoids, far more striking than the conventional type, and varicose veins about the esophagus. Varicose veins of the esophagus are prone to bleed; indeed, this is one of the ways by which cirrhosis kills its victims. The hemorrhage into the gastrointestinal tract may become uncontrollable, and the patient succumbs. Another understandable means by which cirrhosis produces death is through the accumulation of metabolites in the blood that would ordinarily be detoxified or cleared by the liver. These metabolites, such as ammonia, have a serious effect on the central nervous system, and the resulting coma may be the terminal event.

The role of the liver in the metabolism of hormones is also of interest, and the organ's importance becomes evident when it can no longer carry out this role. In the male victim of cirrhosis the testicles tend to undergo atrophy, the breasts enlarge, and there is decreased body hair. In the female, the menstrual periods stop and the breast may either enlarge or become atrophic. If the disease has not reached an established state, virtually all of these findings will reverse with treatment.

The patient does not go from a normal status to advanced cirrhosis overnight. Another of the remarkable features of the liver is its reserve capacity. Although the liver carries out many complex functions and does this 24 hours a day, it was designed in such a way that, if some of the liver cells are damaged or destroyed, there are still cells aplenty that can carry out the required activities of life. This is truly one of the amazing things about virtually all of our vital organs. We can abuse them and misuse them, even destroy them in part, and still have enough left to continue. In fact, we carry on so well that there may be few if any symptoms to warn the person that he has done some irreversible damage to a vital organ. Perhaps we should try to get some word to the master architect of the vital organs that he could improve the next model if a warning system were inserted! It could be extremely valuable if a whistle would blow or a light would flash, so a person could be warned that he had damaged a portion of a vital organ. Under our present system, it is unfortunate that symptoms do not develop until there has been so much damage to an organ that recovery is impossible. It is unfortunate when the first symptoms of liver dysfunction are those of hemorrhage from an esophageal varix. It is equally unfortunate when the first symptoms of pulmonary emphysema occur so late that there are not enough alveoli remaining to reconstruct even a reasonable ease of respiration.

The reasons for consumption of alcohol have nothing to do with the liver. They are much more concerned with the effects on the central nervous system and personal social responses. We will discuss alcoholism at some length shortly; however, here a few comments should be made with reference to alcohol as a food. Certainly, it supplies calories to the body at a greater rate than carbohydrate. Since there is no nitrogen in the alcohol molecule, it cannot be classed as a protein. Chemically, alcohols have a superficial appearance similar to that of carbohydrates; metabolically, however, they are handled more like fats and may be the source of part of the fatty deposition in the liver. Nutritionally, it becomes apparent that alcohol produces calories, but nothing else of metabolic value.* Since there has never been a shortage of calories in the American diet, one must class calories derived from alcohol as wasted or empty calories.

One very important and practical question may be asked in regard to the quantity of alcohol required to produce cirrhosis of the liver. Studies have been reported in the medical literature on this subject. An international symposium held in Sweden in October 1969 was devoted to alcoholic cirrhosis and liver poisoning. A number of studies are reviewed in that symposium. Patient histories of as little as two quarts of hard liquor per month have been associated with evident liver damage. This is especially true if the alcohol is consumed on a daily basis. Patient histories are quite unreliable and usually represent a minimization of the amount of alcohol consumed. There seems to be considerable variability in individual susceptibility to cirrhosis. Obviously, some people are more sensitive to alcohol than others. As mentioned earlier, as few as 10 per cent or as many as 30 per cent of alcoholics develop cirrhosis. The higher figures seem to emanate from the United States. The late progressive effects of liver damage may be interrupted by intercurrent illness, unavailability of alcoholic beverages, or perhaps transitory success in rehabilitation programs. Certainly, any interruption of continuous drinking habits helps to reduce the susceptibility of the liver to cirrhosis. The most classic work on quantitating alcohol ingestion and the development of cirrhosis was done by Pequignot, a Frenchman (1961) and was cited in the above

*7 calories per gram for alcohol.

symposium by G. A. Martini. It is as follows:

1. Borderline for harmless use—less than 80 grams per day. (30 gms = approx. 1 ounce)
2. Risk zone—80 to 160 grams per day.
3. Great risk exists with more than 160 grams per day.

These figures are based on only a 20-year exposure to alcohol. Translated in terms of a 10-per-cent wine or a 5-per-cent beer, this could require one and one-half quarts of beer or one and one-half pints of wine to reach the equivalent of 80 grams of alcohol per day. You may not realize that there is more alcohol in a 12-ounce bottle of 5 per cent beer than in a cocktail containing one ounce of 90 proof liquor. It is assumed that people consuming this quantity of alcohol will also have a normal intake of food. It has been shown that a normal or increased protein intake tends to protect the liver from the effects of alcohol. The reverse is also true. The person who is eating poorly is subject to significantly more liver damage than the person with a regular or excellent diet. In a more recent report in *Preventive Medicine*, Jan De Lint considers consumption of 20 grams of alcohol per day (no time limitation) as characteristic of an alcoholic—no correlation was made with cirrhosis.

Some epidemiological studies of cirrhosis are of interest. In France, Italy, Portugal, and West Germany the death rates from cirrhosis of the liver are approximately twice those in the United States. France is now spending 42 per cent of their health care funds for alcoholism and its related diseases. However, the rate of increase in the United States death rate is higher than in these countries. France is an exception. We may catch up with them yet! On the other hand, Great Britain is showing a decreasing mortality from cirrhosis of the liver. In all countries, the death rate correlates with the amount of alcohol consumed. The decreased consumption in Great Britain is apparently attributable to a high tax on alcohol. Prohibition was not a successful experiment in the United States. However, the death rate from cirrhosis in 1907 was 15 per 100,000. With the advent of prohibition in 1920, the death rate fell rather sharply, and in 1923 was down to 7 per 100,000. It remained at approximately this level until prohibition was repealed and has had a gradual increase since that time and is now back to the 15.5 per 100,000, reported for 1971. A similar phenomenon occurred in Paris. From 1940-45 wine was rationed at .5-1 litre per week. During this period the cirrhosis mortality fell from 35 per 100,000 to 7 per 100,000.

It is not our intent to advise reestablishment of prohibition in the United States on a national level. However, it should be quite apparent that cirrhosis of the liver is a preventable disease and that, even if it does occur but is recognized reasonably early, it is treatable. Once again we have demonstrated that with some medical advice and treatment and the patient's good judgment, a significant number of deaths can be deferred. The government can also play a role in this area, as shown by the British experience. Heavy taxation of alcohol alone may bring about a significant decrease in the incidence of this disease.

Alcoholism

The previous section on cirrhosis of the liver opens the door to a broader discussion of alcoholism. This is a field that is highly charged with social, psychiatric, religious and medical overtones, and many volumes have been written on the subject. When we discuss major causes of death, alcohol presents itself as an enemy in many different guises. Cirrhosis of the liver is a classic example. Our discussion of automobile accidents is another. The vital statistics manual for 1967 listed 2982 total deaths from alcoholism alone. Moreover, another entry entitled "Alcoholic psychosis" accounts for 599 deaths. The role of alcohol in accidents, suicides, homicides, heart disease, gastrointestinal disease, and degenerative brain disorders is not listed, nor can it be obtained from this source. Other sources give rather dramantic statistical information. Chronic alcoholism reduces life expectancy by 12 years. A report from Switzerland states that alcoholism is directly responsible for 3.2 per cent of all male deaths and indirectly responsible for 9.7 per cent of other such deaths as accidents and suicides. Cirrhosis is also increasing in Switzerland. Dr. W. Laurie, director of the state health laboratory services in Perth, Australia, has reported that 3 per cent of all deaths in that country are caused by alcoholism. The Australian data, as well as some data from Chile, indicate that alcohol is responsible for 36 per cent of suicides. We have previously reported the 50 per cent incidence of alcohol involvement in fatal motor vehicle accidents. This figure is confirmed by Australia's experience and is reported to be as high as 74 per cent in Chile. In short, the number of deaths directly and indirectly attributable to alcoholism is impossible to ascertain with any degree of accuracy. However, the number is obviously so very large that it must represent one of the larger groups of deferrable deaths.

The National Institute on Alcohol Abuse and Alcoholism, directed by Dr. Morris E. Chafetz, has submitted a report on alcohol and health to the United States Congress. This is a relatively short and comprehensive, but startling, report. It will serve us as a major reference. Approximately 95 million Americans drink. Ten per cent of these are either alcoholics or alcohol abusers. The cost of alcoholism is tremendous. Ten billion dollars annually is lost in work time. Two billion dollars is required for health and welfare services. Three billion dollars in property damage and medical expenses and other costs result. This makes a total of $15 billion we pay for the privilege of reducing our life expectancy by 12 years. We have tended to consider the alcoholic a problem in character or personality rather than as a victim of treatable illness. We must admit that our medical and psychiatric treatment of cases of alcoholism is less than ideal. However, reports of successful treatment in from 30 to 40 per cent of alcoholics is not unusual. This is a much better success rate than we enjoy with many forms of malignancy, and these statistics could probably be improved with more reinforcement of the attitudes of society in general. Alcohol is truly our nation's most abused drug. This drug is freely accessible and perfectly legal, and it takes far more lives and produces economic loss far in excess of that attributable to illegal drugs.

Prevention of death from alcoholism must be examined from both a short- and a long-range viewpoint. The acute alcoholic is in immediate danger from a number of different mechanisms. Hemorrhage from the esophagus and stomach has already been mentioned. Tears in the esophagus have occurred from vomiting during an acute alcoholic episode. Alcohol may precipitate an attack of acute pancreatitis; in fact, pancreatitis rarely occurs in the nonalcoholic. Even heart failure may result from the direct toxic effect of alcohol on the heart muscle and the associated high volume fluid overload. Pneumonia is common in the acute alcoholic. It is unknown whether this is caused by impairment of the defensive mechanisms of the lung or whether, during a period of inebriation, the patient loses his ability to cough, allowing aspiration of infected material into the lung. All of these very serious and acute complications are treatable by the physician once the patient is present in the emergency ward. Recovery unfortunately does not occur in all cases.

The long-term complications are less dramatic in their onset, but can be equally devastating. We have reviewed cirrhosis of the liver and its associated problems. It should also be added that primary cancer of the liver occurs as a complication of cirrhosis, provided the patient lives at least five years after the cirrhosis has fully developed. Primary cancer of the liver is virtually nonexistent in the American adult who does not have cirrhosis. The central nervous system deterioration leading to personality defects and actual organic psychoses may result from prolonged or chronic use of alcohol.

Our society is filled with paradoxical situations. One of the most striking is our cry for more and better health care while we enjoy and virtually insist upon the use of alcohol in the social and business world. A great deal of our nation's business is transacted with martini in hand. The cocktail party, which is one of the most common urban social events, manifests many of the undesirable features of our drinking habits. It is true that medical care can improve the lot of the alcoholic, but everyone's lot would be much happier if there were no alcoholics. This does not mean that alcohol must be totally abandoned in our society, but it does imply that individuals must use good judgment. If we are to regard alcohol as a socially acceptable psychotropic drug, we need not put up with drunkenness or abuse of alcohol in any form.

Looking Ahead

Almost without exception, when a man reaches his early and mid-thirties, his career plans are established. If he is to be a professional man, most of the time prior to the age of 30 has been spent in academic training. A young man in medicine usually graduates from medical school at the age of 25 or 26. After four years of postgraduate training, he is ready to start his own career. Those of us in medicine frequently feel that we are at a disadvantage by getting a late start. However, other professions and other careers demand equally long periods. Even the businessman or the shopkeeper may require five or ten years before his business can be considered a successful operation.

Women, on the other hand, have a slightly different outlook by the time they have reached their mid-thirties. By her thirty-fifth birthday, a woman has passed the 15th year of the acceptable time for childbearing. Most physicians feel that she should not reproduce after that time, and I have the feeling that most women of that age have reached the same conclusion. At this point, if being reproductive was the most important feature of the woman's career, she may become somewhat depressed, for in this nation of "youth worship" and "glamour above all" she is apt to feel that she has passed her peak. Note then, the contrast that exists between the male in his early 30's and the female of the same age. The male has reached the point of exhilaration; he is just coming into his own professionally. At the same time the female feels that she has passed her peak. It seems at times that the male becomes assertive and confident only as he becomes productive, while the female becomes confident and effervescent only when she is reproductive. Hopefully, as the role of women becomes broader-based, these values will tend to change. Certainly, the decade we have just covered is an exciting one for both men and women. They should enjoy good health. They should be vigorously pursuing their careers. Their families should be started, and their lives should envision ever-expanding horizons. This truly is the first of the decades of duty after the family has been established and a career selected. It is only natural to strive hard for success. It is very common for the man of the house to work long extra hours, perhaps even take a second job or to continue his education with night courses during this decade of striving and scrambling after this nebulous goal we call success.

The foregoing remarks are made only to offer an explanation for some rather obvious happenings in this decade. It is well known among physicians that men in this age group do not come to their doctors for routine checkups or general medical advice. If they are ill, quite ill, they will appear. Otherwise, they are too occupied with the things that are important to them. To the woman, a checkup means visiting her obstetrician to see that everything is all right "down there." Even to her a general medical checkup or general advice is something she regards as more suited to her mother. As a general rule, the children will be taken to the pediatrician for preventive medicine procedures such as immunization and advice concerning nutrition, but neither the father nor the mother thinks of establishing the principles designed to prevent the crippling diseases that will become more evident even in the next decade. Isn't it foolish that we will work so hard for 30 years to achieve success and then take so few steps to prevent its utter collapse by illness and death after a very short time? Whenever a young man with a young family and a budding career is stricken with sudden death, whether by disease or by accident, it causes great sorrow, and people always regret that such a young talent should be lost to society before his time. We all understand that some deaths are unpreventable in all age groups. However, if people did not by their own negligence or their own stupidity throw themselves into the path of the grim reaper, the death rates in these productive years would be considerably lower.

This decade presents an ideal time to institute a number of health maintenance measures. I doubt that a person in this age group needs to have a physical examination each year. However, certainly an occasional examination to record the blood pressure and pulse rate and correct any obvious problems seems warranted for both males and females. Some other general bits of advice include the things we have talked about in previous chapters. By this time the calorie needs of an individual have peaked out and are decreasing each year. This means that weightwatching will be more important than it has been in the past. Dietary habits, therefore, are particularly important. We still insist on a low fat, low cholesterol intake. We have repeatedly commented upon moderation in calories. These precautions must certainly continue. The hazards of alcohol, particularly overindulgence, have just been discussed. Most people, when they enter this age group, have reached the point where they are starting to become sedentary. Athletic endeavors in high school and college age are well behind them. The time demands of their occupation are greater; unless that occupation involves physical activity, all too often it is during this decade that both men and women tend to become slovenly.

This is the ideal age to become involved in a physical fitness program. Some form of physical activity should be followed on a regular basis. Vigorous forms of exercise such as tennis, running, bicycling, and swimming are all much less dangerous to initiate at this age than they are 10 to 20 years later, and their benefits are just as definite now as they will be in decades to come. Proper diet, physical fitness, reasonable self-concern, and the avoidance of bad habits are the key words to the protection of your health and the good life it has taken these thirty-odd years to attain.

XI. The Decade of Danger

Ages 35 Through 44

The duties and responsibilities of the last decade continue in an unrelenting manner through this next ten years. Another ten years of time brings with it a doubling of the mortality rate. The total death rate has now increased to 310.6 per 100,000, and the death rate patterns for the next three decades are becoming apparent. Since the death rate has now increased to slightly over the .3 per cent mark, this period may be described as the first of the decades of danger. The total population in this age group in 1967 was 23,838,000. This represents a slight increase over the last decade. If you wish to find the approximate number of deaths from our death rate charts, the number given on the chart multiplied by 238.4 will give you very nearly the actual number of deaths involved. The causes of death in this decade are indicated in Chart XVI.

It is immediately apparent that a new leading killer is arriving on the scene. Major cardiovascular and renal disease is the leading cause of death for the first time in the decade between ages 35 and 44. From now on, this will be the leading cause of death; its role as a killer will become more apparent with each decade. At this point, we need to break down this term and identify its component parts. When we say major cardiovascular and renal disease, we are really saying that there is an interrelationship between the heart, the blood vessels, and the kidneys. Everyone understands that there is a relationship between the first two; however, the addition of renal disease to this complex may be confusing. A certain number of renal diseases either produce or are the result of heart and vascular diseases. For instance, we know that if the blood supply to one kidney is reduced because of abnormality of a blood vessel leading to that kidney, that kidney will give off a toxic substance that will elevate the patient's blood pressure; this, in turn, may overload the heart. With this interrelationship we have demonstrated how the blood vessel may result in damage to the kidney and how the kidney in turn damages the heart. Another mechanism by which the interrelationship can be demonstrated involves kidney disease of a primary type such as glomerulonephritis. Glomerulonephritis is a descriptive term by which we say that a certain portion of the kidney is involved in a disease process that lowers the efficiency of the organ. This may be an infectious process or it may be a so-called autoimmune disease—a sensitivity reaction to some substance within the patient's own body or some reaction of unknown origin. With this initial or primary type of kidney abnormality, again, toxic materials in the blood increase, and the blood pressure elevates. With the elevation in blood pressure, the heart may be damaged; alternatively, some of the blood vessels may be damaged and the patient may have a stroke, which is a rupture of blood vessels in the brain. Once again, we have demonstrated the interrelationship of the heart, the great vessels, and the kidneys. Not all kidney disease is involved in this relationship; therefore, not all kidney diseases are listed in this category. For instance, polycystic disease of the kidneys and congenital deformities are not included; neither are infectious disease of the kidney and obstruction to the urinary outflow. These entities at the moment are included in the diseases not listed among the top 60; possibly they appear under infections or birth defects.

Since this is the first decade in which major cardiovascular and renal disease becomes the leading killer, I feel that it is worthwhile to break down the death rate from each of these component parts of this disease complex. The heart disease portion of the complex creates mortality figures as follows:

> Rheumatic heart disease, 6.0
> Arteriosclerotic, degenerative, and coronary heart disease, 55.5
> Hypertensive heart disease, 5.0
> Other, 5.3
> Total, 71.8

Obviously, the heart disease component of this complex is the largest, and coronary heart disease with its arteriosclerotic and degenerative manifestations forms the big portion of the heart disease group. We can point out from our chart that more people are now dying from coronary heart disease and arteriosclerotic changes than are killed by accidents. This component of major cardiovascular and renal disease alone kills nearly as many persons as malignant disease in this age group; as I have implied, it will become a larger and larger factor in our mortality figures in each future decade.

Vascular disease breaks down into the following components:

> Vascular disease of the central nervous system (strokes), 15.4
> Generalized arterial disease, 0.2
> Peripheral manifestations of hypertension, 2.5
> Other generalized vascular disease, 5.1
> Total, 23.2

The central-nervous-system type deaths are rather clearly defined and represent strokes of one type or another. Other complications of hypertension are less well known. Hemorrhages can occur from any vessel, and one of the most dramatic is that from the aorta. If hypertension has existed for some time, it is perfectly possible for the aorta to rupture; this is a dramatic cause of death. I must also state that aneurysm of the aorta with rupture can occur in nonhypertensive patients. Generalized arteriosclerosis is a relatively unusual disease in this age group, but does warrant an incidence of 0.2. Other vascular diseases are usually of the autoimmune type, already described, such as lupus or a diffuse type of arterial reactive disease such as polyarteritis nodosa.

The renal component of our major syndrome is relatively small, particularly in this decade; our statistics manual lists 3.4 as the incidence under this component portion of the symptom complex. The rate of death from major cardiorenal disease increased by slightly more than four times in this decade compared to the one previous.

Malignancy becomes the number two killer in our current decade. It increased by slightly less than fourfold over the decade earlier. The incidence of malignancy is 60.3 per 100,000. In more exact numbers, malignancy took the lives of 14,384 people in this age group in 1967. Since our numbers are becoming so large, it is becoming more and more reasonable to use death rate figures rather than actual numbers. Since we are dealing with a large number of deaths, it also seems reasonable that we should offer you a breakdown of the types of malignancies that occur at this time. The pattern has changed a great deal from that seen in the teen-age period. The pattern to be presented here is similar to that which will exist through the coming decades, although some changes will develop. The following represents the type of malignancies and the mortality rate distribution in this decade:

Oral cavity, 1.1
Digestive, 10.8
Respiratory system, 10.0
Breast, 10.5
Genital, 8.8
Urinary system, 1.4
Leukemia and lymphoma, 4.9
Other, 9.9
Total, 57.4

Females suffer more from malignant disease in this age group than males. The relative ratio is 68 females to 52 males; 57 per cent of the total are female. This sex relation is primarily caused by the difference in incidence of cancer of the breast and cancer of the female genital system compared to comparable organ systems in the male. Fortunately, both carcinoma of the breast and carcinoma of the cervix, which are the leading cause of death from malignancy in females, are decreasing as killers. Improvement in figures for cancer of the cervix is dramatic; the figures for breast malignancy improve only slightly. This is primarily the result of improvement in medical treatment and improved early diagnosis.

Accidents remain in the number three spot as a killer in this decade. In looking over the distribution and types of accidents, it appears that they do not change remarkably from the previous decade. Some increase in incidence of accidents on the job is noted. Deaths in motor vehicle accidents are down slightly. Deaths from accidental falls are somewhat increased.

As predicted in the previous chapter, the incidence of deaths from cirrhosis of the liver has increased. It has increased slightly more than fourfold from the previous decade.

Infectious disease has taken an increase in this decade

for no obvious reason. In reviewing the details of death from infection in this period, all infectious processes seem to show a modest increase in occurrence. This is especially true in pneumonia, where the incidence has doubled over the previous decade. The incidence of homicide continues to decrease. Suicide continues to increase, although the changes from the previous decade are reasonably small.

You will note that we are still carrying deaths from complications of pregnancy. In this decade, they are down to 1.1. However, remember that this death rate is based on the entire population of this age group and not in respect to the number of deliveries. The incidence of death complications has fallen from 1.6 in the previous decade to 1.1 in this decade. However, to put this statistical information in its proper perspective, you need to know the number of live children born by mothers in each decade. Women between the ages of 35 and 44 delivered 294,376 babies in 1967. In the same year, women between the ages of 25 and 34 delivered 1,306,799 babies. Therefore, our 0.5 drop in mortality figures occurred in a population that delivered over a million fewer babies than in the earlier decade. This emphasizes the point made previously, that pregnancy in females over the age of 35 shows an increased risk to the mother; further, as we have emphasized, it is a considerably greater risk to the infant. This reiterates our earlier contention that good reproductive health exists only between the ages of 20 and 35.

Under category number seven, we continue to carry a number of entities, well known to most people, that produce relatively few deaths. However, from this group we have extracted diabetes, and hereafter we will identify it as a separate entry. Diabetes takes lives throughout the entire age spectrum. From this point on, primary adult diabetes will be listed as a separate entity. Its mortality rate is relatively low in this decade, but it will increase as the decades pass.

Pulmonary disease other than infection or neoplasia involves primarily bronchitis and emphysema. This had a very low mortality in the last decade, but has increased about fourfold since that time. It, too, will increase strikingly in the decades to come.

Birth defects, of course, now take relatively few lives, but this entry persists throughout life and is not limited to the first decade. For this reason we have continued to carry it through each chapter.

Fundamentals of the Heart

In 1628, William Harvey published his work on the circulation of the blood. Since that time every student has learned that blood enters the heart by the right atrium and passes from there through the tricuspid valve into the right ventricle. From the right ventricle, it is pumped through the pulmonary valve into the pulmonary artery and into the lungs, where the blood is oxygenated. Blood returns to the heart by means of the pulmonary veins and enters the left atrium. From the left atrium it goes through the mitral valve into the left ventricle and is pumped from that ventricle through the aortic valve into the aorta and to the systemic circulation. This system consists of large arteries and increasingly smaller arteries, down to capillaries that perfuse the tissue; the blood passes through the capillaries into small veins, then into larger veins, and subsequently enters the superior vena cava and returns to the right atrium. Although this pattern of circulation has been accepted since the 1600's, our information concerning the details of each step along this trip has increased manyfold since that time.

Throughout the preceding pages of this book, I have repeatedly recommended a diet modest in calories and low in fats and cholestrol. I have repeatedly suggested the adoption of some type of physical fitness program. I have inveighed against smoking. I have warned against obesity and elevated blood pressure. These cautions were designed to decrease the risk of your having a heart attack. This advice is not unique. You have read this in magazines and perhaps in books. To be meaningful, advice must be explained. To explain the advice we have offered, and will continue to offer, we will give only fundamental information. This includes physiology, its alterations, and meaningful statistical data. We have given you many statistics and will continue to do so. The data offered have come from the most fundamental sources I can locate. These sources have been primarily United States Government statistics and world medical literature. In discussing the physiology of the heart, I would like to approach it from the viewpoint of its three different components: the electric circuitry, the muscle itself, and the blood supply or nourishment of that muscle. Obviously, these are all interrelated, but as we speak of heart attacks, sudden death, and heart muscle damage, we will allude to the various component parts involved.

Muscles contract following electric stimulation from nerves. This is especially true of skeletal muscle. The impulse originates in the central nervous system and travels to the muscle. The stimulated muscle contracts to move the arm or leg or other appendage. The central nervous system exerts modest control on the cardiac muscle. Certainly, it can increase the heart rate. The heart muscle is unique in that it can initiate its own beat and can also control its own rhythm. The heart of any animal removed from the body will continue to beat so long as nourishment is provided to the muscle. Obviously, the electric stimulus that forces the muscle to contract must have its primary origin within the heart itself. Regardless of how this control originates, there is a recognized pathway by which impulses travel to stimulate the muscle of the heart. Chart XVII shows the basic conduction pattern of the heart. Impulses originate in the normal heart at the sinoatrial node (SA node). This node is high in the right atrium and, because of its position, it can monitor the blood returning to the heart. If there is a sudden increase in blood supply coming into the heart, impulses can be fired more rapidly, and the heart rate increases. On the other hand, if the patient is at rest and the venous return is slow, the heart can take advantage of this and reduce its rate. Regardless of this pattern of changing stimuli, the impulses begin at the SA node. From here they spread in a radial manner throughout the surface of the right atrium and extend through the interatrial myocardial band into the left atrial wall. Since the speed of the impulse through the atria is relatively fast, the atria contract, for all practical purposes, simultaneously. The impulses tend to be gathered or returned to the atrial ventricular node (AV node). This node is in the posterior right side of the septum separating the right and left atria. Once gathered here, the impulses are conducted through a common pathway (the bundle of His) to the interventricular septum, where they divide, one series of fibers extending along the left ventricular side, the other along the right ventricular side. Fortunately, the conduction time through the AV node and the bundle of His is increased slightly so that the ventricles can be effectively filled by the atrial contractions before they themselves contract. As the impulse extends over the right and left bundle branches extending toward the ventricles, the first area of the ventricles to become excited is the interventricular septum. The wave of activation spreads into the substance of the septum from both the right and left bundle branches. The early contraction of the septum makes it rigid and allows it to serve as an anchor for the contraction of the remaining ventricular heart muscle. The endocardial or inner surfaces of both ventricles are activated rapidly. The impulse extends from the inner surface to the outer surface, and the ventricles contract promptly.

Following contraction, there is a refractory period which means that the heart will not accept stimuli for a short time, thus permitting the electric system to repolarize and the heart muscle to prepare for its next contraction. This refractory period serves, under normal circumstances, to maintain the rhythm of the heart.

Unfortunately, there are times when the normal rhythm is not maintained. Changes in the cardiac rhythm can be the result of a block any place along the conduction system we have described. Changes in rhythm may result from the origin of an impulse outside the usual SA node. Any portion of the heart has the potential of initiating an electric impulse. Under normal circumstances, this does not occur; if it does occur, it is to be hoped that it is only a temporary situation. Most people at some time in their life experience premature contractions of the heart. In most instances this is an entity of little clinical significance and is probably caused by a stimulus arising from some portion of the heart other than the SA node shortly after the refractory period. The best clinical description of what happens from the standpoint of the individual is that there is a feeling that the heart flops over in the chest. When the heart beats at a normal rhythm, we are unaware of its action. When the premature contraction occurs, a strange feeling in the chest results. The premature contraction is usually followed by a prolonged diastolic period, following which normal rhythm recurs. If premature contractions become frequent, they can be annoying to the patient and usually imply some additional irritability of the heart, but in themselves are relatively benign.

Under certain conditions, the cardiac muscle undergoes an extremely irregular type of contraction that is quite ineffectual in propelling blood. Such an arrhythmia is called fibrillation. It may involve either the atria or the ventricles. Atrial fibrillation usually results from some chronic type of heart disease, most commonly rheumatic fever and its involvement of the mitral valve. When this occurs, there is a continuous uncoordinated-type contraction of the auricles, and these contractions contribute little to ventricular filling. Ventricular filling becomes irregular, and the impulse to contract the ventricle is basically dependent on those impulses that reach the AV node and to lesser extent dependent upon the stretching of the ventricular muscle fibers. Therefore the ventricular rate is also an irregular one. Atrial fibrillation is an inefficient type of cardiac activity, but it is quite compatible with life and even with reasonably normal activity. Ventricular fibrillation is a considerably different entity. This results in rapid loss of consciousness and usually death within a very few minutes. The ventricles contract in an uncoordinated and continuous manner, and there is, for all practical purposes, no output of blood from the ventricle.

The mechanism of the production of ventricular fibrillation is explained by two different theories. One states that there is a continuous radial or circus type impulse in which the cardiac action is stimulated continuously and there is a breakdown in the refractory period. The other theory holds that the impulses are discharged at relatively high frequency from several different ectopic areas in the atria and ventricles. The result is the same; the heart musculature is under continuous fire to contract. The contraction either follows a very short refractory period or breaks through that refractory period completely.

It is possible to treat patients with atrial fibrillation by means of drugs. The treatment of ventricular fibrillation is a much more dramatic process, since this activity is totally incompatible with life. Patients can be salvaged by applying electric current directly to the chest wall. This shocks the heart and permits the reestablishment of a normal cardiac rhythm. The electrical stimulations can be used on patients with atrial fibrillations or other dysrhythmia. The electrical correction of rhythmic disorders is referred to as cardioversion.

The heart is a pump, and its design is a very simple one. The chambers of the heart are separated by means of septa (walls) and valves that open and close at appropriate times and under appropriate stimulation. The amount of work that the heart accomplishes during the course of a person's lifetime is truly tremendous. Like other vital organs that we have mentioned, the heart exhibits a remarkable reserve. When at rest, it functions in a leisurely way, yet under stress or stimulation it can respond with heroic efforts.

A few comments in reference to heart valves seem appropriate. Heart valves consist primarily of thin flexible flaps of fibrous tissue that are attached to the base of a very sturdy fibrous ring. The action of the valve leaflets is primarily a passive one; like any other valve, its function is to maintain a unidirectional flow of the blood. There are two general types of heart valves. One type is the totally intracardiac valve that rests between the auricles and ventricles. The valve between the right atrium and right ventricle is the tricuspid valve. The valve between the left atrium and left ventricle is the mitral valve. When speaking of valves in general, these two are included together and referred to as the atrioventricular valves. They are somewhat different from the other paired valves in that they have strong muscular filaments attached to the free edge that lead down to the papillary muscles that arise from the ventricular walls. These muscles contract at the same time as the ventricle contracts, therefore helping to hold the valve closed and preventing it from being everted by the ventricular systole. The aortic and pulmonary valves are more simple in their operation. They have no muscular attachment. When the ventricle contracts and raises the pressure of the blood within that chamber, the valve is passively opened. When the ventricle is empty and the ventricle starts to reexpand or relax, the pressure in the vessel peripheral to the valve becomes higher than that within the ventricular chamber, and the valve is forced to close. During ventricular systole, the cusps of the valves do not go all the way back to the wall of the vessel, for some eddy currents develop between the valve and the vessel wall. This is particularly important in the aortic valve; if the valve cusps were to open completely and lie against the aortic wall, they would block the openings of the coronary vessels.

All heart valves tend to be subject to two general types of abnormality. If the valve ring is too large and the cusps do not come together in such a way that the lumen is completely obliterated, the valve is said to be insufficient. On the other hand, if the valve ring is too small or the cusps are too stiff and impede the exit of blood from the given chamber, the valve is said to be stenotic. It is also possible that a valve may in part be stenotic and at the same time not close efficiently and therefore be insufficient. Such valves are said to have combination defects.

The heart muscle itself has been studied in great detail. Even so, there are a number of things that we do not understand about it. It certainly has many similarities to ordinary skeletal muscle and yet, as we have implied, it has the power within it to stimulate its own contraction and to maintain its own rhythm. This is indeed unique. This capacity for self-stimulation and self-control has led to the theory that there are electrochemical changes at the cellular level that are responsible for this type of behavior. Three chemical elements are known to be involved. These are sodium, calcium, and potassium. Their presence in proper proportion and their shift across the cell membrane into and out of the extracellular space presumably generate the electric energy needed for continuous heart stimulation. It is known that calcium tends to produce contraction of the heart and that potassium tends to inhibit contraction or relax the heart. It is also known that, without sodium, neither of the calcium or potassium effects can be produced, and that the potassium level within the cell tends to be higher than in the extracellular fluid, while the other ions tend to be in closer equilibrium. All of these studies imply that an electrochemical process actively taking place at the heart muscle cell level requires ions that must be maintained in proper balance.

Other physiological properties of heart muscle deserve comment. The ability of tissue to respond to stimulus is referred to as excitability or irritability. The degree of irritability may vary from time to time, depending upon the chemical or nervous environment in which the cell finds itself. We know that heart response or muscle contractability tends to be an all-or-nothing response. At any given moment, depending upon the irritability of the heart, the minimal stimulus that the heart muscle will accept will result in a maximal contraction. A more vigorous stimulus, therefore, does not invoke a more violent response. The amount of stimulation required to produce the contraction will vary from time to time and depends upon the irritability of the heart.

The changes of increased irritability are interrelated with the discussions previously given involving abnormal cardiac rhythms. Certainly, if the heart muscle is in a nonirritable state, small ectopic stimuli from areas other than the SA node cannot produce a premature contraction or a dysrhythmic contraction. On the other hand, if the heart is in an excitable or irritable state, small ectopic stimuli may very well result in abnormal rhythms. Therefore, chemicals or drugs that alter the heart irritability become extremely important to us.

Another mechanism by which the heart changes its rate

and force of contraction is described basically as Starling's law. This law states that, when a muscle fiber is stretched, it will be stimulated to contract. There are, of course, reasonable limits that must be established, for gross overloading or overstretching results in tear of the muscle. All muscle tends to respond according to this rule. The heart itself is a perfect example. You will recall that the SA node is close to the entrance of the superior vena cava. As the blood flow from the superior vena cava is increased, the right atrium becomes slightly more distended than previously, and contraction is brought on more promptly. The same is true of the ventricle. As the ventricle is stretched, it is stimulated by the filling process itself and therefore reacts with added vigor to the internal electric stimulus. It is by means of this physiological process that the heart controls its rate to meet the demands of the moment. Physical exercise increases the stroke volume and the pulse rate; as a result, there is an increase in the volume pumped per minute. As the heart rate increases up to 120 beats per minute, the amount of time the heart spends in contraction does not change a great deal. The period the heart has for diastole is shortened as the pulse rate increases. If the venous return is increasing, the amount of time needed in diastole for chamber filling is also decreased. Once again, the system works very effectively.

One other significant difference between cardiac and skeletal muscle needs to be mentioned. Skeletal muscle can work hard for short periods of time under repetive and sustained contraction. In this way it will use up more oxygen than is actually supplied. In other words, skeletal muscle can build up a substantial oxygen deficit. In contrast, cardiac muscle is required to contract repetitively for a lifetime and is quite incapable of surviving significant oxygen debt. For this reason, the blood supply to the heart muscle itself must be very rich, and the substances necessary to supply the heart with oxygen and food must be readily available. To do this, a very rich capillary supply is provided in the heart; approximately one capillary is noted per fiber. In this manner, the diffusion distances for oxygen and carbon dioxide are short and the gases are carried in and out with dispatch. Any suggestion of oxygen debt is a strong stimulant to the heart. At this point we are ready to discuss the major factors controlling the blood supply to the heart muscle itself. Chart XVIII shows the gross coronary circulation.

As we have implied, heart function is critically dependent upon the amount of oxygen and food materials carried to the cardiac muscle through the coronary circulation. This does have some unique features but, in general, it is governed by the same laws that govern the flow of liquid through any form of tube. The flow of liquid through any tube is dependent upon the diameter of the tube, the pressure difference between the two ends of the tube, and the resistance encountered in the tube itself.

Man has two major coronary arteries. Each arises in the lower portion of the aorta, respectively behind the anterior and left posterior cusps of the aortic valve. These two vessels supply the entire blood flow to the heart muscle. The right coronary artery supplies the right atrium and right ventricle. The left coronary artery supplies principally the left ventricle and the left atrium. The right coronary artery is dominant in approximately 50 per cent of individuals, the left coronary artery is dominant in approximately 20 per cent. The dominant artery supplies the diaphragmatic wall of the left ventricle. The flow delivered by each vessel is equal in the remaining 30 per cent. Total coronary blood flow should be expressed specifically in cubic centimeters (cc) per minute per hundred grams of heart muscle. After the blood passes through the capillary beds of the heart, it returns by venous channels through the coronary sinus and into the right atrium. Some accessory venous channels are present, but these are of little importance.

If one were to measure the amount of blood flowing through the coronary arteries as the cardiac cycle progresses, it would become evident that, with ventricular contraction, the extraluminal pressure on the coronary vessel becomes so great that blood flow in the proximal portion of the coronary arteries, especially the left, is actually reversed. The flow on the right may not be so clearly reversed, since the right ventricular contracting muscle volume is smaller than on the left. As soon as the end of systole is reached, the heart muscle starts to relax, the aortic valves close, and perfusion through the coronary vessels is markedly increased. Therefore, most of the perfusion that occurs in the coronary vessels takes place in diastole. It is evident that, other conditions remaining the same, as the patient develops tachycardia (rapid rate) coronary perfusion decreases moderately; as the heart rate slows, coronary perfusion is moderately increased. If there were physical factors only, perfusion would be markedly increased during diastole compared to systole. However, with the development of tachycardia, the heart uses more oxygen and more glucose, and the metabolic by-products developed tend to lower the resistance of the peripheral myocardial vessels. In this way there is a compensatory factor for tachycardia, especially when the tachycardia is the result of increased muscular exercise. Several other terms and concepts are important if we are to understand the work load of the heart and the adaptations that the coronary circulation and the myocardium must make in order to permit the heart to carry out its wide variation in total work load. The volume of blood propelled from the left ventricle with each contraction is referred to as the stroke volume. The minute volume is the stroke volume times the pulse rate. The amount of work done by the heart is the stroke volume times the arterial pressure. One could theoretically double the stroke volume and halve the peripheral pressure, and the amount of work being done would be the same in both instances. The quantity of blood being ejected with each beat from the left ventricle in the average healthy man at rest is between 60 and 70 cc. An equal quantity of blood is discharged at the same time from the right ventricle, making a total cardiac output of 120 to 140 cc. The contents of the left ventricle are ejected against a much higher pressure than are the contents of the right ventricle, since the pressure of the pulmonary artery is only approximately one sixth that of the aorta. The minute volume is usually expressed in terms of one ventricle. The amount of work done by the left ventricle is obviously considerably more than that done by the right ventricle. In consequence, the left ventricle is usually the thicker, heavier, and more muscular of the two.

It is evident that the heart can increase its output per minute by increasing its stroke volume and maintaining a constant rate or by maintaining a constant stroke volume and increasing its rate. Frequently, both factors are increased when the demand is large. However, since the time required for the heart to contract is relatively constant (0.3 seconds up to the rate of 120), any increase in rate must be made at the sacrifice of diastolic filling. It is also reasonable to assume and scientifically proven that there comes a time when increased heart rate can no longer increase the minute volume. If only slight shortening of the systolic period can be obtained and if we were to triple the pulse rate, it would become apparent that there would be practically no time left for diastole. If diastole is short, there will be inadequate filling of the ventricular chambers, and the stroke volume will by necessity fall. Of course, if the pulse rate approaches a threefold increase, there must be some shortening of the systolic period. Even with reasonable shortening of the systolic period, the diastolic period is too short to allow adequate ventricular filling.

Under the simulus of stress, whether it be muscular exercise or emotional stress, the oxygen consumption of the heart, because of its increased work, may be increased by a factor of as much as eight to ten. Since we cannot possibly increase cardiac output by means of increasing heart rate by more than threefold, other means of increasing oxygen utilization must be available. It is at times of stress, as we are implying here, that cardiac minute volume is modestly increased within the limits of the short diastolic period. The oxygen demand of the heart is met by increased coronary flow. The muscular metabolites lower vascular resistance, and at the same time the coronary vessels dilate. Increasing the diameter of vessels is the most efficient way of increasing blood flow through that vessel. This is the mechanism by which the heart survives periods of stress.

For coronary perfusion of the myocardium, ideally we would like to have vessels of a large caliber that could supply more blood than is actually needed. We would prefer that the cardiac rate be slow, therefore, providing excellent perfusion during the period of diastole. We would also like to see overlap between the major or collateral vessels develop between the right and left coronary arteries, thus offering some protection against small vessel occlusion. We also want the coronary vessels to be elastic. We prefer the heart muscle not be irritable so that extopic stimuli will not result in abnormalities in heart rhythm. These are the desirable physiological goals we will try to achieve.

The Arteries and Their Diseases

In our preceding section, we discussed the heart at some length, and in this discussion it should be apparent that the arteries are a direct extension of the heart. The heart must depend upon the coronary arteries for its oxygen and fuel. At the same time, the heart is pumping blood to the peripheral tissues to supply oxygen and fuel for their needs. The vessels carrying the blood from the heart to the tissues are considerably more than conduits. Primarily, one describes the artery as elastic. If one examines an artery in cross section, one notes that there are three general layers. The inner lining is a smooth, slick surface referred to as the intima. The middle layer, the media, is actually a muscular tissue that provides both resistance and elasticity. The outer layer is a loosely but firmly woven fibrous layer referred to as the adventitia. The inner layer, the intima, is smooth and designed to keep friction of the flowing blood minimal.

As the heart ejects its stroke volume, the intraarterial blood volume increases; since the arteries are elastic, the volume of the vessels increases. At the end of systole, the aortic valve closes, and the pressure within the aorta and great vessels tends to maintain a constant steady perfusion into the small arterioles and capillaries. Thus, the elasticity of the vascular bed changes the pulsating flow of the major arteries to a steady stream in the small peripheral vessels. If the peripheral resistance is low, the pressure within the great vessels is also relatively low, and perfusion continues without difficulty. If there is high resistance in the peripheral tissues, the pressure within the great vessels remains elevated, and the next systolic ejection of the heart must take place against a remaining pressure load. This pressure within the great vessels is referred to as the blood pressure. When patients have high blood pressure, referred to as hypertension, it is apparent that the heart must work against this elevated resistance. This is a significant problem, for it increases the work load of the heart, it increases its oxygen consumption, and it results in enlargement of the heart secondary to this high pressure. If the heart enlarges, there will definitely be a problem of supplying the additional heart muscle with blood through the coronary vessels. We defined coronary blood flow as the number of cubic centimeters of blood per 100 grams of heart muscle per minute. With increased heart mass, we immediately have a reduction in coronary flow.

The peripheral arterial bed has another unique feature that differentiates it from any other pipeline. Since it has muscle within its wall and since it is a part of living tissue, it responds to chemical or nervous stimuli, and this response will be one of either contraction or relaxation within the wall of the vessel. It is therefore possible for a local vessel to identify a need and respond to it. This is clearly evident when an area of infection starts in the skin. One can actually see the redness and swelling that occur over the site of the insult. The blood vessels have been told that there is need for additional blood supply to this area, the arterials have responded by dilating, and preferential blood flow goes to the area where it is needed. This works in many different ways. When one is exercising the arms, the blood supply to this area will be increased because of local metabolic needs. Blood can be supplied on demand to a local area if the demand and needs are greater than usually provided. Examples of infection and work are those that result in dilatation of the local vascular tree. If, on the other hand, cold is applied to the skin, the vessels contract, in this way protecting the blood from significant decrease in temperature and the body from heat loss. All of the functions that I have attributed to the vessels, depend upon one thing: the vessel must remain elastic.

We are now ready to discuss some of the diseases that occur to blood vessels. They are of two types: localized and generalized diseases. The localized diseases will be discussed only very briefly. The most obvious, of course, is trauma, with rupture or tearing of a vessel. This usually, but not always, requires medical assistance in order to prevent excessive hemorrhage. When such an event occurs, the vessel immediately goes into contraction in an attempt to stop hemorrhage; if the vessel is small enough, it may succeed. On other occasions, the ruptured artery may actually be adjacent to a ruptured vein and the two may mix their vascular contents at the site of injury and eventually heal in such a way that the blood mixes between artery and vein. This is referred to as a traumatic arteriovenus fistula. Another local form of arterial disease is an aneurysm. This is simply an abnormal bulging or dilatation of a vessel that results from a weakness in its wall. The arteries constantly carry a pressure load. This load varies from second to second; if a weak spot is present in an arterial wall, a bulging or ballooning of the vessel may occur at this point. This is, of course, very dangerous, since rupture is the logical terminal event. We also know that local vascular disease can occur peripherally. This implies narrowing of these blood vessels as they go to the periphery. This may be a part of generalized vascular disease; in some instances, only the blood vessels of the legs may be involved. Here again, the vessel loses its elasticity and tends to be narrow in caliber. The results are poor blood supply to the feet or involved area. The final results depend upon how severely the arteries are involved. In some instances this may result only in uncomfortable or "cold feet." In other instances, it may be more severe and result in inability to walk or run, while in the most extreme degree, the blood supply to the feet may be lost, resulting in gangrene, requiring amputation.

There are several forms of diffuse arterial disease. However, from the standpoint of mortality figures, only one is important. This is arteriosclerosis, referred to as hardening of the arteries, and this clearly describes the physiological barrier that this disease process entails. The arteries lose their normal elasticity. Since all of the services the arteries perform are dependent upon the elasticity of the vessel, this is a serious disease. Since it occurs with increasing incidence in older populations, it is regarded as a degenerative disease or a disease process of aging. I am not certain that this is entirely true. From a physiological standpoint, the reverse may be the case. One of the most characteristic features of premature aging is vascular disease. The function of virtually every organ is dependent upon its blood supply. If that supply could be maintained at youthful levels into older age periods, it may well be that the process of aging could be considerably retarded. Rather than thinking of arteriosclerosis as a process of aging, I offer the concept that aging is the result of arteriosclerosis. I will of course, admit that processes other than arteriosclerosis are involved in aging, but maintaining a good blood supply to all vital organs would do more to stop the aging process than any other process. I have referred to arteriosclerosis as a diffuse disease. This is not entirely true. Certainly, in advanced cases when all of the vessels are badly damaged, to the radiologist as he examines the X ray films or to the pathologist as he examines the specimens it appears that arteriosclerosis is a generalized disease. However, apparently in the beginning, arteriosclerosis starts in a localized area, the atheroma. It may start in several different localized areas simultaneously, but these patches may be quite far apart and may represent, again, only local manifestations of disease rather than diffuse involvement of the entire arterial bed as the term "hardening of the arteries" implies.

It is obviously and unfortunately impossible to study the evolution of arteriosclerosis in a given person from a very young age until he is very old. It is not feasible to look at the inside of arteries without removing them; once removed, they can no longer be studied in longitudinal fashion. Therefore, all of the research on arteriosclerosis has been done by observing material in different age groups within a given population or by comparing different populations of the same age group to each other. The first lesion that is evident within a major artery is a "fatty streak." This fat exists around the cells of the intima of the vessel and may actually be inside the cells of some of the defending white cells in the area—the macrophages. This fatty material is predominantly cholesterol. The earliest lesions occur in the aorta and can be observed in infancy. By the age of ten, virtually every American child demonstrates fatty streaks in his aorta. By the time a person is 25 years of age, some 30 to 50 per cent of the aorta may exhibit fatty streaks.

The time required for these soft, fatty streaks to convert to more dense fibrous tissue (atheroma) is not known. Neither is it understood why these lesions tend to be localized. It may be that the hemodynamic forces and the arterial wall stresses are part of the reason. These factors also play a role in the conversion from the fatty deposit to the more fibrotic atheroma. We also know that these plaques tend to increase in size. The method by which the plaques grow (atherosclerosis) apparently is related to continuous and progressive fat or lipid accumulation from the blood. This mechanism may be the same as that which initially generated the fatty streak. As our atheromatous plaque, which is now a mixture of fibrous tissue and fat, becomes larger, it obviously produces an obstruction to the flow of blood. As the plaque increases in size, additional complicating factors may occur. For instance, there may be slight tearing around the margin of the plaque caused by hemodynamic forces. Blood can become trapped within the plaque. This blood clots; this in itself increases the size of the plaque and eventually serves as a hard calcific nidus as part of the healing process. This calcification with its scarring and stiffening of the arterial wall is arteriosclerosis. The amount of blood flow impairment that results from our plaque depends upon the percentage of the vessel lumen that is narrowed by its presence.

There is evidence to suggest that the fatty streaks and even the fibrous plaques that are accumulating more fatty material are reversible. This information must come from animal studies. It has been studied in the monkey, which is considered most comparable to the human for evaluating disease processes. To my knowledge, there is no evidence, once hemorrhage, ulceration, calcification, and scarring have occurred in the plaque, that reversibility of the disease process is possible. Because the end-product lesions of arteriosclerosis are quite irreversible, I have heard many of my professional colleagues state that preventive measures after the age of 30 are fruitless. Don't you believe it! Atheromatous plaques are continuously progressing to arteriosclerosis. Fatty streaks are starting every week throughout the entire spectrum of life, and each of these streaks may well go through its evolution to an ulcerated hard plaque described above. It is perfectly evident to all of us that there is far more arteriosclerosis in the 80-year-old than in the 40-year-old person. It is difficult to say with scientific certainty that, had preventive measures been instituted at age 40, the end point would be different, but certainly all logic implies that this is true. Every plumber knows that the pipe gets rusty because of the content of the liquid it carries within. High cholesterol blood levels imply many fatty streaks and large fibrous fatty atherometa.* We would like to prevent that cholesterol level from ever rising over 175; this is why our advice at the end of the first year of life was to reduce the cholesterol intake. This is obviously the time at which dietary control should be initiated. However, at the same time, if new plaques are being laid down or started later in life and there is evidence to point toward reversibility of the lesions, lowering the cholesterol blood level would seem like a good health measure at any age.

A study from Finland is reported in *The Lancet* for October 1972. Finnish physicians took advantage of the long-term hospital stay of mental patients. Two hospitals were involved. One hospital substituted a cholesterol-lowering

*Dr. William E. Connor of the University of Iowa has stated that, if the serum cholesterol never rose beyond 180, no one would ever die of arterosclerotic disease.

diet for the regular hospital diet, the other hospital remained on a regular diet. After a six-year period, the diets of the two hospitals were reversed. Twelve years after the start of the study and with 29,217 patient years of data, the results are being published. In men the mortality from coronary heart disease was cut to one half by the special diet in both hospitals. In the hospital where the age group was highest, women also enjoyed the same improvement. In younger women there was improvement, but it was not statistically significant. We have known for many years that women prior to menopause enjoy partial protection from arteriosclerosis and coronary heart disease. We now have definite evidence that lowering the serum cholesterol levels can reduce coronary heart disease mortality in middle-aged adults.

The points where these plaques form is extremely important. Obviously, a small plaque in the center of the large vessel such as the aorta will produce little or no physiological handicap. True, there will be some roughening of the aorta and perhaps some alteration of blood flow at that point. This will be undetectable. However, if this small plaque has its point of formation in a vessel that is relatively small and leads to a critical portion of the brain, one can easily imagine that there may be alteration in the brain's ability to perform its duties. The same is true when a plaque develops in the coronary vessel; there will be a decrease in the amount of blood that can flow to the heart itself. There is apparently some hemodynamic stimulus that determines where these plaques form. They occur frequently at the places where vessels branch. This is unfortunate, since it narrows the opening of the artery and reduces the amount of blood that can enter it. We mentioned earlier some of the relationships between vascular disease in the kidney and resulting heart problems. The arteries that lead to the kidneys arise from the aorta at virtually right angles. This type of angulation seems to offer a favorable point for the formation of atheromatous plaques. It is by these means that renal blood flow may be reduced and changes in kidney function result. The same can be said for other organs, but it is most critical in the areas of the kidneys, brain, and heart. Other evidence of hemodynamic forces lies in the fact that these plaques are not seen in the pulmonary artery unless there is elevated pulmonary pressure. Since that pressure is normally about one sixth of that in the aorta, it would seem that there is some relationship here. Certainly, the fat content of the blood in the lung is the same as that in the aorta and on the left ventricular side of the circulation. Therefore, not only is the blood cholesterol level important, but the patient's blood pressure is also very important in speeding up or slowing down the arteriosclerotic process.

It is appropriate that we discuss hypertension, or high blood pressure, in this section as a part of arterial disease. We have already implied that the blood pressure present is related to the resistance of the small vessels peripherally. This implied that hypertension was a peripheral vascular disease. In a sense, this is true. Certainly as the peripheral vessels become constricted and offer more resistance, the blood pressure elevates. This does not give us a clue as to why the peripheral resistance increases. There are a number of instances in which the etiology of this peripheral resistance can be determined; however, there are others in which it remains unknown. As we have mentioned before, there are times when substances released by an hypoxic kidney will result in high blood pressure. There are also times at which hypertension can be related to tumors of the adrenal gland. However there still remain some 80 to 90 per cent of cases with hypertension the etiology of which is unknown. This does not mean that there is no treatment for hypertension. Medication has been used very effectively for long-term management and has been reasonably successful.

The important thing to be remembered from this short

discussion is that, primarily, hypertension represents another significant risk in the development of coronary heart disease, and even more importantly that it is a risk for which there is reasonable medical treatment. The long-term medical management of hypertension has been successful; with the control of hypertension, this risk factor of coronary heart disease is decreased. The diastolic blood pressure, which normally runs between 75 and 85, if raised to over 105, increases the risk of major myocardial infarction by a factor of four. Therefore, elevation of diastolic blood pressure, in the same manner as elevation of blood cholesterol, represents a risk factor in the development of coronary heart disease.

In addition to the increased incidence of heart disease, every study indicates that strokes and cerebral vascular accidents are closely associated with hypertension and, in fact, are probably more closely aligned with hypertension than any other single entity. The medical profession has long recognized the fact that the sudden cerebral accident, or stroke, is more common in the patient with chronic high blood pressure. We have referred to the significance of diastolic blood pressure; however, if calculations are based on elevation of systolic pressure, findings are much the same. Diastolic pressure has been reported here because this was the portion of hypertension reported by the National Task Force on Arteriosclerosis. This report is relatively recent in its publication, and fortunately for our purposes, also uses the year 1967 for evaluation. Physiologists have also reported to us that the diastolic pressure is the best evidence of peripheral vascular resistance. The systolic pressure simply implies the force with which the heart must act in order to overcome the resistance of that peripheral force and to inject the stroke volume into this semiexpansive space, the arteriovascular tree.

One of the concerns of physiologists and physicians for

many years has been the relationship of salt intake to the development of hypertension. We have commented in previous sections that the infant should be encouraged to eat a relatively low salt diet, and that infants do not crave the same amount of salt as many adults. Part of this is a matter of training and education. Most of us could live with a considerably lower intake of salt than we now accept. It is felt that lowering the salt intake may well play a role in reducing the number of hypertensive patients in our population. Some recent reports have challenged this long-standing hypothesis. Be that as it may, we know that, if hypertension can be identified clinically and treated medically, the patient will improve and that this risk factor can be controlled. Certainly, this is one of the reasons for recommending a periodic physical examination. This examination need not be an extensive one; if all findings are normal, the physician can best advise you as to when the next examination should be scheduled. Hypertension is a significant finding and should always be noted. Even relatively minimal amounts of hypertension are now considered so significant that medical treatment is immediately instituted.

In summary, the arteries are an extremely important organ system. There arteriosclerosis starts, develops, and becomes a problem. Small arteries are structures that offer resistance to the blood flow and therefore result in high blood pressure. Arteriosclerosis and hypertension are primary factors in coronary heart disease; every step should be taken both medically and from the standpoint of health maintenance to keep these two factors at a minimum.

Myocardial Infarction

(Heart Attacks)

The broad category of cardiovascular diseases accounts for over half of the deaths in the United States in 1967; see Appendix, Chart XXXII. This chart is copied from the bulletin of the National Task Force on Arteriosclerosis. Its figures have been checked against the *Vital Statistics Manual* of the United States 1967 (mortality) Vol. 2 Part A and are certainly valid. Of those 625,850 deaths caused by arteriosclerotic and degenerative heart disease, 412,027 were attributed directly to myocardial infarction—death of heart muscle because of reduced oxygen supply. The remaining 213,823 are the results of complications of either arteriosclerotic heart disease or myocardial infarction. (Heart failure several months or years after infarction.)

There is no way of knowing how many people in this country suffer myocardial infarctions (heart attacks) each year. It is well known to the medical profession that a number of myocardial infarctions are asymptomatic. It is only at a later date, when electrocardiographic studies are done, that the evidence of scarring is detected in the heart itself. The patient can give no history of symptoms that might be related to the objective finding. We therefore conclude that a significant number of myocardial infarctions are small; because the heart's reserve is great, the patient continues to function and experiences no immediate difficulty.

In our previous sections we have implied that there are various ways in which the heart can be damaged when its blood supply is less than its need. Of those deaths that occur secondary to acute myocardial infarction, approximately 50 per cent occur within the first hour. Some of these occur in a matter of minutes. This makes up the group commonly referred to as "sudden death from myocardial infarction"; a recent article says that it is nearer 60 per cent. There are no entries in *Vital Statistics* identifying the number of victims who die a sudden death; a conservative estimate would be 200,000 per year. There is virtually no way these victims can survive. If it were possible to have a hospital within eight blocks of every person in the entire country and if it were possible to have coronary intensive care units in every one of these hospitals, we would still do little about reducing the death rate of this group. Even the currently popular emergency care system teams would have trouble getting to the proper address in a short enough period of time to make a real reduction in death rate in this group. A study from Edinburgh indicates that more time is spent by the patient trying to decide whether he should call his physician or attempt to go to the hospital than it takes to get to the hospital once the decision is made. The average patient takes approximately two hours to make up his mind that the symptoms are significant and to seek medical aid. This is, of course, too late for the 200,000 people we have mentioned above. Therefore, for 200,000 people per year, myocardial infarction must be prevented or it will continue to be buried—I mean this literally—just as we have done over the past decades.

If a patient arrives at the hospital, he has statistically eliminated himself from this very high risk group. The mortality statistics of the hospital-admitted patient with myocardial infarction are rather encouraging. The mortality rate is approximately 15 per cent of the admitted patients. This has improved because of constant monitoring in intensive-care units and prompt treatment of rhythm disorders. Among patients admitted, the largest number of deaths occur from "cardiogenic shock." This occurs when such a large segment of the heart muscle is damaged that the heart, as a forceful pump, cannot maintain an adequate blood pressure, and death results. Some work now being done in the field of heart-support systems is encouraging. On occasions, surgery may be helpful to this group of patients. Even so, this represents a considerably smaller number of patients than those in the sudden death category. There are other causes of death during the period of hospitalization. These are very important to the physician, but not very important to us. They include rupture of the heart; rupture of the papillary muscle that results in eversion of a heart valve;

heart failure because of a loss of overall cardiac muscle; additional clot formation within the coronary vessel, resulting in more extensive heart infarction; and late-developing arrhythmias that occur as a complication of the healing process. We should mention that, during this period of recovery, cardiologists are careful not to let the patient's pulse rate become too slow. This is in contrast to the advice we have given in this text. However, this is an abnormal situation. During the period of recovery from myocardial infarction, if the heart rate drops into the low 50's, the long diastolic period may result in ectopic beats. This is not desirable, and protection against arrhythmias of all types is considered paramount during this period. This is so important that, if the pulse rate gets in this low range, a pacemaker may be used to bring the rate to more satisfactory levels.

If the patient survives the acute heart attack and the period of hospitalization, statistics indicate that his five-year mortality rate is in the area of 28 to 30 per cent. We can show very clearly that myocardial infarction is not a totally disastrous disease simply by pointing to the statistics. We all know patients who have had myocardial infarctions and have lived normal lives for many years. Even so, every patient who has had a myocardial infarction would be better off had he not experienced that disease. Medical care is encouraging. The surgical techniques being used to increase the myocardial blood flow are indeed exciting, and they would seem to offer hope for decreasing the mortality rate for this disease entity.

These operations are designed to by-pass a narrow segment of a coronary artery. The usual operation is to take a vein from the leg and connect one end to the aorta and the other to the coronary artery beyond the area of narrowing. This is very effective initially, but the arterial pressure soon has a telling effect on the transplanted vein. The vein wall thickens in response to the pressure; after two years some by-pass grafts have obliterated. Those two years may be important in reestablishing heart circulation and function, but basically the coronary by-pass is a palliative procedure. The use of an arterial segment for the by-pass may be more successful than the use of a vein, but technically this is not always possible.

These operations represent a form of preventive medicine, since patients can be treated before a disastrous event occurs. There is no surgical technique available that can compare in efficiency to preventing the disease in the first place.

Before starting a specific discussion on the prevention of myocardial infarction, some additional comments on heart muscle injury are indicated. A popular magazine recently reported that all heart attacks were caused by stress. I will accept this, provided you will give me a liberal definition of stress. Stress can occur as a result of strenuous physical exercise when the oxygen demand of the heart muscle is greater than that which can be supplied by the stiff coronary circulation. The same type of stress can occur from a vigorous emotional stimulus. Certainly, the heart muscle is grossly stressed if a clot forms and occludes a coronary vessel. This can occur even with a normal vessel. Worries and irritations are emotional stresses. These stimulate the adrenal glands to increase the production of adrenalin. This in turn may produce damage to the heart muscle directly or simply increase the heart rate. No one can accurately evaluate the role that emotional stress plays in the incidence of coronary heart disease, but clinicians in practice imply that it is a significant factor. It is of some interest that, in the Framingham study, marital difficulty, principally divorce, did not seem to act as a significant risk factor.

Most emotional responses such as anger and fear result in increased heart rate. This is considered to be a generalized response to adrenalin. It has been suggested that there are also some focal effects of adrenalin or other endocrine substances on the heart muscle that might be produced under emotional stimulus. These can result in focal or even microscopic areas of heart damage. As a result of this, the circulation in this small area will be sluggish, and additional clots may form. This results in a progressive form of myocardial infarction. At any time during the development of such a process, local chemical changes can occur. This specifically results in loss of potassium from the myocardial cell, and this alters the electrochemical generator that we have previously described. With chemical changes, ectopic stimuli may arise from these focal areas, and arrhythmias such as fibrillation may result. This is certainly one of the mechanisms of sudden death and one that can occur without significant arteriosclerosis. On the other hand, if the heart muscle is not irritable and the area involved is relatively small, the patient may have no symptoms. A great deal depends upon the irritability or susceptibility of the myocardium and the extent of the initial damage.

If the changes we have described above can occur in people who have normal coronary vessels, certainly they can also occur with even greater frequency in patients who have coronary artery disease with reduced flow. Hard, rigid vessels can dilate very little, so their ability to supply oxygen to the heart muscle on demand is quite poor. Patients who have coronary artery disease of the arteriosclerotic type have one advantage over the patients with no coronary involvement; this advantage lies in the fact that arteriosclerotic narrowing in a coronary vessel develops as a slow process. Therefore, the heart muscle has a limited chance to compensate for these slow changes. It is known that the greatest stimulus for the development of collateral circulation is the presence of an arteriosclerotic plaque in the coronary vessel. Therefore, if a plaque develops in the vessel and if it grows slowly, it is possible that other vessels may increase the blood supply to the risk area. Such collateral circulation does not occur unless it develops under some form of stimulus.

It should be evident at this point that there is no single cause for myocardial infarction, but many causes. It is also apparent that myocardial infarction does not always produce death; it may not even produce symptoms. Prompt availability of good medical care offers moderate hope for improving mortality for myocardial infarction, but by far the greatest hope lies in an active program for preventing this disease.

Prevention of Myocardial Infarction

Since myocardial infarction can result from a number of different mechanisms, no single approach to prevent it is adequate. If we are to make a significant reduction in the number of deaths occurring from coronary heart disease, we need to instigate measures that will improve our odds in the following categories.

1. Prevent arteriosclerosis by keeping the coronary vessels large and elastic.

2. Reduce the myocardial irritability so that stimuli arising from areas other than the SA node will not result in erratic myocardial contractions. This comes with increased myocardial efficiency.

3. Maintain a relatively slow pulse rate at rest. In this way acute stimuli that double or triple the heart rate will not throw the heart into an impossible situation in maintaining cardiac output and coronary blood flow.

4. Hypertension must not be permitted to go unchecked. This is primarily the physician's task, but there are

things the patient can do; certainly, he must present himself to the physician before the blood pressure can be identified.

5. Social and psychological stress must be identified.

When we say that we wish to institute a program to prevent arteriosclerosis, this is an ambitious statement. Arteriosclerosis is our major contemporary medical problem. It is the process associated with aging. At this point, no one has a magic bullet that will knock it out. Neither do I expect anyone to develop one within the foreseeable future. All of our risk factors involve the development of atherosclerosis. However, a low serum cholesterol level is the best insurance in our arsenal against arteriosclerosis. A low cholesterol can be obtained by various means. We know that countries that do not indulge themselves in the high fat diet we in the United States enjoy do not suffer high death rates from arteriosclerosis and coronary heart disease.

The level of cholesterol in the blood is considered an indicator of coronary heart disease risk. Control of the serum cholesterol level may be considerably more complex than just making the minor dietary adjustments we have mentioned. An elevated cholesterol may be the result of liver, kidney, or thyroid disease, and no reduction of the serum level can be accomplished until these diseases are corrected. There are well recognized genetic differences in cholesterol metabolism. If you are fortunate enough to belong to a genetically determined group that can eat anything and maintain a normal cholesterol level, you are fortunate. On the other hand there are persons who maintain a very high cholesterol level on standard food intakes. These persons require long-term diet planning and frequent serum cholesterol determinations. It may be that their cholesterol level will not drop until other dietary adjustments are made. Restrictions on sugar and saturated fat may be needed before cholesterol levels will fall. Drugs may be used in severe and resistant cases. The interelationship between sugar and cholesterol is interesting, but not completely understood. Diabetics show higher cholesterol levels than nondiabetics. Reduced consumption of simple sugars and alcohol may lower cholesterol. We know that simple sugars in the presence of insulin enter the fat cells and form triglycerides. Triglycerides are a form of fat; no one is surprised that we can make fat from sugar. These triglycerides are thought to be atherogenic, and their level in the blood tends to follow but does not necessarily parallel the cholesterol level. While we do not definitely know the relationship between triglyceride and cholesterol metabolism, triglycerides may be precursors of cholesterol. We know that some hypercholesterolemia is carbohydrate- or sugar-dependent. However, lowering the ingestion of cholesterol and saturated fats is generally the most effective way of lowering the cholesterol level. If this modest dietary manipulation fails to lower the cholesterol, a more detailed study of circulating fats will be required.

Therefore we may say the serum cholesterol level can be lowered in several ways. The following are well-established methods.

1. Reduce cholesterol ingestion.

2. Increased ratio of polyunsaturated fatty acids to saturated fatty acids in diet.

3. Significant weight reduction.

4. Long-term vigorous exercise programs.

5. Medications designed to involve the cholesterol-bile salt cycle.

The American Heart Association has gone on record as recommending that no one should have a diet of over 300 mg of cholesterol a day. This is a stringent reduction from the average American diet. Certainly, the average American diet contains at least twice that much cholesterol and there is no doubt that many people in this country have diets in excess of 1000 mg of cholesterol a day. One can control the amount of cholesterol ingested per day easily, provided that one eats his meals at home and the family has given some thought to the maintenance of a reasonable diet. However, when one eats at a restaurant, it is virtually impossible to maintain this level of cholesterol intake. This is especially true of our gourmet restaurants. I have witnessed people consume as much as a half pound of butter in one meal. Can you imagine lobster, corn on the cob, and fresh bread being eaten without copious amounts of butter? I would like to point out that this gourmet meal with the half pound of butter could be consumed with less than two pats. Lobster is very good with lemon juice and a dash of salt. Fresh bread needs no spread of any type to add cholesterol and calories. If one must have something to spread on bread, jelly, honey, preserves or corn oil margarine can be substituted. I must admit that corn on the cob does require a small amount of butter or corn oil margarine, but certainly not a copious amount. This same person may very well have enjoyed eggs, bacon, toast with butter, and coffee with cream for breakfast. His lunch may have been a cheeseburger and malt with or without French fries. How's that for the one-day diet of our successful American business man?

It is not my intention to fill this text with recipes or diets. There are many books available on the low-fat, low-cholesterol diet. The cholesterol contents of some selected foods are listed in Chart XXXIII in the Appendix. The very few simple rules we have indicated all along the way make it impossible for anyone to overindulge himself on a high cholesterol diet that so many people seem to enjoy. These rules include an avoidance of egg yolk, whole milk, butter, and ice cream and cheese made with whole milk. In their place one uses corn oil margarine for butter, sherbert and fruits for desserts, skim milk in place of whole milk, and egg substitutes. These rules alone will keep you in a reasonable cholesterol diet range.

The American Heart Association recipe book published by John McKay should be a valuable addition to any home library. In addition, an egg substitute is available. Standard Brands has introduced "Egg Beaters," a cholesterol-free egg substitute; its protein, vitamin, and mineral content is very close to that of eggs, but it is essentially cholesterol-free. This is progress. The Australians have also shown that they can improve the saturated-polyunsaturated fat ratio and lower the cholesterol content of beef by altering the diet of cattle. More progress.

This organization of the kitchen should begin early in marriage. It should be taught to the children at a very early age, and they should grow up appreciating the food that has a low fat content. The earlier in life this type of diet control can be started, the better. This is why our recommendation is to start reducing fat intake at the end of the first year. However, since most of us did not start at age one, we should not throw up our hands and say it is impossible. Atherosclerosis to arteriosclerosis is a progressive diease. It is our suggestion that everyone have a serum cholesterol determination, if it is under 175, it may not be necessary to have it repeated on an annual basis, and diet restrictions become of minor importance. However, if it is over 175, dietary measures should be taken immediately to see that it be returned to this general range. The strictness of one's diet can be controlled by the level of serum cholesterol.

One of my internist friends disagrees with this philosophy. He feels that a serum cholesterol determination is unnecessary, for all of us should live and eat as though our cholesterol level were high. His point is well taken. I have accepted a cholesterol level of 175 as a safe level; it is not as safe as a level of 120, which is the level maintained by most Japanese. It is, however, safer than 250, which is the level so many Americans carry and call normal. I am sure that most students of coronary heart disease epidemiology would be delighted if the average American cholesterol level could be reduced to 175. It is therefore apparent that the 175 cholesterol level I ask you to strive for is possibly short of ideal—but it is indeed an improvement and may be difficult to achieve.

If we can keep the cholesterol level down, this risk factor in the development of coronary heart disease is minimized. At the same time, we may be keeping vessels to the brain and kidney open and pliable and slowing the aging process. Everything is to be gained. So, while prevention of coronary heart disease is our major objective at this time, the means by which we accomplish this achieve many other purposes.

Another benefit that comes from the low-fat, low-cholesterol diet is its relative ease of weight control. It is possible to get enough calories in the form of carbohydrates and protein to gain weight, but it is much easier to gain weight if a high fat diet is maintained. This is true because the body gets approximately 9 usable calories per gram of fat compared to 4 in carbohydrate and protein. We have in general said very little about obesity as a risk factor for heart disease. There is some evidence to suggest that obesity alone does not increase the risk of myocardial infarction unless it exceeds 25 per cent over normal. However obesity is usually accompanied by hypertension and elevated blood cholesterol. These are the factors that are definite risks to the heart. Obesity is a risk in many other ways. Certainly it is a social problem.

The second means by which we are attempting to reduce deaths by myocardial infraction is by reducing myocardial irritability. It is difficult to find many specific means in this area. However, there are many implications. Some are based on clinical grounds, and others are based on the laboratory findings. One means of reducing myocardial irritability that can be demonstrated in the laboratory and in clinical practice involves the relationship of tobacco and heart disease. Nicotine can be shown to increase the irritability of the heart. Clinically, this is borne out by the increased incidence of sudden death among smokers. At least eight of ten persons who die suddenly from myocardial infarction are cigarette smokers. One reference states that 97.5 per cent of the victims of fatal heart attacks in men under 50 are smokers! Apparently, the smoker maintains a nicotine and carbon monoxide level in the blood high enough to increase heart irritability. In addition to creating irritability, the carbon monoxide of the smoke combines with the hemoglobin to make it less efficient in carrying oxygen and it also increases the tendency for clots to increase in size. This compounds the problem. These features alone are enough to make sudden death from myocardial infarction virtually a smoker's disease.

Other drugs may influence the irritability of the heart muscle. Digitalis, a life-saving drug in cases of heart failure, may be dangerous if used improperly. Caffeine is also a stimulant and may very well affect heart irritability. The Framingham study showed no coronary risk in drinking up to five cups of coffee per day. A more recent report from the Boston Collaborative Drug Surveillance group indicates that there is an increased risk if over five cups per day are consumed, and the risk is dose-related. There are some doubts about the Boston study. They may not have completely separated coffee from coffee and cigarettes. If you are a heavy coffee drinker you may experience irregular heart beats—premature ventricular beats. Reducing coffee consumption alone may correct this irregularity. Keeping one's coffee consumption under five cups per day should impose no great hardship, and it may be very important in reducing heart irritability.

Myocardial irritability can be reduced in other ways. We believe this change occurs with physical fitness programs. There is some evidence that the numbers of premature contractions decrease rather strikingly as one proceeds in a physical fitness program. Actually, as the heart becomes conditioned, many of the central nervous system and adrenal stimuli are counteracted. This point has been made by Dr. Wilhelm Raab in his book *Preventive Myocardiology,* published by Charles Thomas, 1970. He is a strong advocate of the endocrine route of mediation of the central nervous system and the emotional problems that result in myocardial infarction. As the heart muscle is physically trained, it contracts sharply and more efficiently; as a result, the refractory period is increased and, we believe, irritability of the heart is also decreased. In this way the adrenogenic stimuli from the nervous system are counteracted by physical fitness.

Scientifically acceptable data that physicial conditioning reduces myocardial irritability in the living, intact human are hard to find. Our best evidence is related to dysrhythmias; even persons who have had a myocardial infarct have fewer premature beats if they are on a tolerable exercise program.

If we can maintain a slow resting pulse rate, the heart is protected by several different mechanisms. First of all, the nervous stimuli mentioned above or any other internal drugs are not breaking through to result in tachycardia.

Keeping the pulse rate slow results in more adequate perfusion of the coronary vessels during the long diastolic period. In addition, when adverse or strong stimulation reaches the heart, it will respond efficiently. We have stated previously that no one can survive a heart rate over 200 for any prolonged period of time. It is possible that the heart rate can double or triple under given stimulation. If the resting pulse rate is 60, and the pulse rate is tripled, it is still a tolerable 180. If the pulse rate is 80, and it is tripled, it is an intolerable 240, and the person cannot survive for a very long period. Such stimuli can occur in life. Let me give an example. Let us assume that our example is a vigorous, healthy male in his middle years who has just met a very attractive female. After a short period of time, he finds her flirting quite exciting. As a result, his pulse rate goes up slightly, possibly 50 per cent, which in itself is not very remarkable. Let us assume that nature proceeds along the natural path and our gentleman takes this female home one evening and visits her in her apartment. During the course of the evening, events are moving well, and one exciting event leads to another. At this point, there is little doubt that our hero's pulse rate has doubled. Now let us assume that things are going very well and that an emotional or possibly even a physical climax is approaching. Then the door opens, and her husband arrives on the scene. What happens to the pulse rate now? There is already a double resting rate; very likely it would be stimulated to triple. Whether our hero escapes or not may very well depend upon what his resting pulse rate was before this started. Three times 60 equals 180; he would survive. At three times 80 or 240, our lady's husband needs no gun. This example, with its sexual implications, is realistic. Extramarital sex has resulted in a significant number of myocardial infarctions. Postinfarction patients are especially advised to avoid extramarital affairs. There are many other examples one might quote that would be less dramatic. Emotional trauma in driving through traffic, irritating phone calls, and recurrent bills. We are all subject to many stimuli that bring our pulse rate to dangerous levels. How dangerous depends on how well trained our heart is before the stimulus arrives. Physicial conditioning acquired by exercise programs permits us to tolerate these many stresses successfully for an exercise program is a series of controlled stress periods directed toward improved heart function—thus safety.

Does physical fitness truly protect against myocardial infarction? Certainly, my remarks have implied that this is the case. Those of us who are enthusiastic about physical fitness must guard against losing our scientific objectivity. Controlled experiment is the scientific method of choice. This is often impossible when dealing with humans. The next best method is to establish steps or rules for gathering statistical data so that they are scientifically meaningful. At this point let me introduce you to the steps that are necessary to prove causal, or in this case, beneficial relationships between a factor we are evaluating and a disease process. These same steps are applicable to smoking, hypertension, elevated cholesterol levels, or any other risk factor in myocardial infarction. They apply to bacteria and disease or carcinogens and cancer. Some situations make the criteria hard to meet, but this does not denigrate the system. Keep this system in mind, not only as you read this book, but as you read other claims of great discoveries in the medical field.

1. Logic. The relationship of the factor and the disease must have some initial physiological logic. For example, a snowfall in the Alps should have no logical relationship to myocardial infarction in the United States. In contrast, the risk factors listed previously would pass this step. This step is the least important of the scientific steps, for even if a wild assumption passed here, it would soon fail as subsequent steps were met.

2. Dose relationship. The greater and more prolonged the exposure to the factor, the greater the risk of the disease in a given population.

3. Epidemiology. The distribution of the disease must be the same as the distribution of the factor.

4. Therapeutic trial. Removal or reduction of the factor for a given population must result in a reduced incidence of the disease within a certain period of time.

As you review the steps and think of the risk factors, it is clear that cigarette smoking and hypertension clear all steps with an overage of data at all levels. Cholesterol as a risk clears all steps to 4. Step 4 has been a difficult one for advocates of cholesterol risk to clear. The first data to clear this step were referred to earlier in the Finnish report of diet control in mental hospitals. These are extremely important data; a great deal more data of similar type are expected over the next five years. These data will come from both the United States and Europe.

To establish an inverse relationship between exercise and myocardial infarction is the next consideration. There is no question concerning the logic of the relationship. There are countless books and articles discussing the relationship of exercise and myocardial infarction. The question of epidemiology is answered by the Framingham studies and at least 14 similar studies. These studies support the increased incidence of coronary heart disease in the sedentary. Even the critics of the benefits of exercise will pass in favor of this relationship. Steps 2 and 4 are harder; they are related in this instance. How can we quantify exercise or sedentary living? Some definitions can be offered and are helpful; they may need revision with time. A sedentary person is one whose job requires little physical activity and who has no planned exercise program. He is a sports spectator, not a participant. At the other extreme, Dr. J. N. Morris, a highly respected British investigator, has defined vigorous exercise as exercise that burns 7.5 calories per minute—450 calories per hour—continuing uninterruptedly for 30 minutes. Moderate exercise is defined as 4 to 7.5 calories per minute for 30 minutes, and light exercise is less than 4 calories per minute, with no restriction on time. Chart XXXV in the Appendix gives some examples.

As we define degrees of energy expended as exercise, we begin to find groups of people in whom we can define the incidence of myocardial infarction and in this way check for a dose relationship. The data are incomplete, but there is now enough information available to establish a trend. Dr. T. Bassler reports that no marathon runner has ever died of a myocardial infarct. This is a small number of persons compared to our total population, but it represents a significant sample when compared to the high incidence of myocardial infarct in the general population.

We have previously referred to Dr. Morris' definition of vigorous exercise. He is the principal investigator in a very important article appearing in *The Lancet* for February 17, 1973 that deals with exercise as a preventive of mortality from coronary heart disease. The mortality of myocardial infarction clearly decreases as exercise intensity increases. He evaluated only the leisure-time activity of men with sedentary jobs. His study included 16,882 middle-aged males over a two-year period. This study adds strong data for scientific steps 2 and 3.

Step 4 requires that persons at risk be relieved of that hazard by introduction of the factor—in this case, exercise. The above references are encouraging, but critics will say that anyone who can exercise to this degree may be genetically or metabolically different from the rest of the population. We doubt this, but other studies are appearing.

Start with a group of men who have already had a myocardial infarct; after they recover, put part on exercise programs and treat the others in the traditional way. This is being done in the United States and in Europe. Reports will be more complete in another two years. At the moment, results statistically favor the exercise group, but the trend is not as overwhelming as we would like. One feature of the American study (*Journal of the American Medical Association,* March 5, 1973) is fewer premature ventricular beats in groups of patients in exercise programs, and this in turn reduced mortality. The Swedish physicians are somewhat further into their studies than the Americans. They too are cautiously optimistic. Physicians, especially researchers, are a conservative group, but a pattern has nevertheless developed. Sedentary men are high risk; moderate levels of activity, especially leisure time activity, reduce risk; marathoners run virtually no risk; and even the highest risks of all (those that have had previous infarcts) enjoy reduced mortality with exercise. I am satisfied that physical conditioning reduces risk of mortality from myocardial infarction.

Hypertension is primarily a medical problem. This is one of the reasons for the initial checkup and for following the physician's advice in terms of subsequent examinations. Significant hypertension at least triples the risk of coronary heart disease; certainly, it increases the work load on the heart, causing the muscle to enlarge without significant increase in blood flow. This in turn results in a reduction of blood per gram of heart muscle. There are many ways of treating hypertension; since this is determined individually, no specific treatment will be recommended here.

Certain psychological, sociological, and behavioral factors have been shown to be associated with increased risk of coronary disease. It is assumed that they mediate their influence through the adrenal gland or the central nervous system, as we have described. However, it is very difficult to evaluate emotional stresses and the role they may play in creating a risk factor. In an attempt to be logical in this area, the National Task Force on Arteriosclerosis attempted to divide these emotional factors into predisposing and precipitating types. The predisposing factors include major changes in the cultural environment. An example might be moving to a new country, moving from the farm to the city, or totally changing one's career. This would produce long-term insecurity, which might also come under the large umbrella term "stress." In the same set of categories, a certain overt type of behavior is described as "coronary prone." The coronary prone personality has been defined as including extremes of competitiveness, agressiveness, haste, impatience and recklessness. One specific personality trait attributed to the coronary personality relates to conversation. When you converse with him, he tends to finish your sentences. He listens so intently and is so involved that he predicts the discussion and cannot contain himself. As one looks over this list, it is easy to see why it is difficult to form any kind of quantitative estimate as to the significance of these risks. Dr. Meyer Friedman has written an entire book on personality and coronary risk. Type A personality, which includes most productive people, is coronary-prone. Type B is less susceptible. However, all of the extensive heart studies such as the Framingham study were done on quantitative findings, and their data apply to all personalities.

Under the category of precipitating events, we would include such more common stresses as "loss of a loved one," "loss of a job," "severe financial reversal," or the "breakup of a love relationship." Other workers have implicated overwork and a feeling of intense job responsibility as being precipitating factors in coronary disease. Life dissatisfactions are more frequent in coronary-type persons than in other groups.

Most people react to the problems in a style relatively characteristic to themselves, but quite differently than another person who might be subject to the same stresses. In looking over the literature in this area, one cannot help but be impressed by the many unsolved problems. The social scientists may be of help to us in identifying potential coronary heart disease patients, but more standardized techniques of collecting and studying the data will be required.

It is apparent that we have described multiple risk factors in the development of coronary heart disease. They have included an elevated serum cholesterol, elevated blood pressure, the use of cigarettes, and a lack of physical activity. Chart XIX represents the combination of risk factors as determined by the National Task Force on Arteriosclerosis. The chart is designed for men age 30-59. This evaluates only three of the risks we have defined. The Framingham project has also evaluated the risk of sedentary life and has shown that those people tend to have an incidence of coronary heart disease two to three times as great as the active person. No hard data are available comparing all four risks that we have mentioned. However, as one looks at the chart it seems that, with the addition of each risk, one approximately doubles the mortality rate. We would therefore estimate that, by adding the fourth factor of sedentary life, the combination of all four risks would raise the mortality rate to around 320 to 340 per 1000.

A number of other risks could also be included. We have already mentioned the risk of personality and psychosocial circumstances. Psychosocial pressure therefore can be a fifth risk. Personality is a difficult thing to change. Each individual can take certain steps to minimize the psychological and social pressures we have mentioned previously, and more certainly if they are identified. There is no way for most of us to return to the rural life of our ancestors, but by recognizing the fact that life in the city or suburbs brings a certain amount of social and financial pressure, we can make some adjustments. One may tend to arrange his life style in such a way that the biological impact is minimized.

We can also add obesity as a sixth risk factor, although obesity without other accompanying complications is not as great a risk as an elevated cholesterol or the three major risks. By the time they reach their 40's, both men and women tend to be overweight. By the time women pass the menopause, it is estimated that at least 40 per cent are in the range of being 25 per cent overweight. This factor, plus the fact that an elevated estrogen level seems to protect the arteries from arteriosclerosis, probably accounts for the increased incidence of myocardial infarction in females over the age of 50.

As we mentioned before, diabetics can certainly be added as a seventh risk. Vascular disease of all types is aggravated by diabetes. I prefer to think that an elevated blood sugar either on a prolonged or intermittent basis increases atherosclerosis. The mechanism of this most probably involves increased serum triglycerides and cholesterol. Assuming this broad role of sugar and atherosclerosis enables us to offer preventive measures. The diabetic must be well controlled. Even the nondiabetic should avoid loads of simple sugar. Complex carbohydrates are good and necessary foods, but one should avoid loads of simple sugars that rapidly elevate blood sugar levels.

Our society is based on freedom of choice. However, it seems that in such a society there should be information on the effects of that choice. Even without the addition of the fourth risk factor, sedentary living, the fifth risk, personality and psychosocial problems, the sixth risk, obesity, or the seventh risk, elevated blood sugar, the chart is rather impressive in its evidence concerning development of coronary heart disease. The person who maintains a low serum cholesterol and a normal blood pressure, does not smoke, and is a reasonably active individual has a low incidence of coronary heart disease.

In addition, there is evidence to suggest that there are protective physiological processes. See Chart XX. This embodies the Framingham data that show fewer heart attacks in people with slow pulse rates and a good vital capacity. These are the by-products of physical conditioning. I cannot tell you whether both a slow pulse and a good vital capacity occurred in the same persons and if both are needed to reduce the coronary risk, or if each process is protective. I discussed this with Dr. William Kannel of the Framingham project; he feels his data can not answer this question, but he also feels that a poor or decreasing vital capacity is dangerous. This physiological condition probably is involved in both the sedentary life and smoking risks. If you find it important to your ego to violate all of the risk factors, there is no question that you can push your chances of having myocardial infarction by the age of 60 up to the 90 per cent mark. In this way you can be assured that you will live no longer now, despite good available medical care, than you would have lived had you reached age 60 in the days of the Roman Empire. On the other hand, with none of the original three major risks our Chart XIX shows the incidence of major coronary events to be 20 per 1000.

If the Framingham data as shown in Chart XX are applicable, we may reduce the 20/1000 to 5/1000 by maintaining a pulse rate of less than 67 and vital capacity greater than 3000; for women, the latter figure would be 2300.

It is on the basis of these risk factors and our ability to manipulate them that we say that most myocardial infarctions are preventable. Would you prefer to be in the group with 0.5 per cent risk or the group with 90 per cent risk of myocardial infarction? The choice is yours.

The Program For Physical Fitness

The idea of the physical fitness program repels most men of my generation. Our experiences with physical fitness programs in our younger years were related to military experience, high school athletics, or to proclamations telling us that to be physically fit was an obligation to our country. Physical fitness as preparation for athletic events or for active duty in the military had a certain degree of logic. However, for those of us in noncombat roles, calisthenics and drilling under the stimulus of patriotism seemed somewhat illogical. Those of us who were active in high school or college athletics recalled in subsequent years that we felt better during that time when we were "in shape"; as a result, we sporadically participated in conditioning games. However, most people did like my roommate in medical school, who used to quote Mark Twain to the effect that whenever he felt the urge to exercise, he would lie down and take a nap until that feeling went away. This attitude was certainly prevalent among adults in the early 50's. Those who maintained any type of physical fitness from that time until now were certainly the exception to the rule. We are now in our late 40's or early 50's. Signs of aging are beginning to appear; with this comes a certain amount of boredom and mental fatigue. As a result, one tends to develop anxieties and to become somewhat oversensitive about decreasing physical adeptness. Caloric needs are decreasing, but we tend to overeat and overdrink, which in turn adds to the vicious circle.

Had physical fitness been presented to us in our early years as a means by which we would feel better, accomplish more, and face life more aggressively, our interest might have been greater. Had we been told at that stage in life of the high risk of coronary heart disease and that physical conditioning might improve our odds against that disease, I believe we would have been better motivated to participate in such a program. Even if we had been told that it was a program for improving our "zest for living" and if we had been given other more selfish reasons, such as maintaining a more attractive physique, the program would have been much more appealing.

Books and articles that are written for the public, as well as those written for the medical profession, now offer various attractive incentives for physical conditioning. I am a strong believer that it plays a vital role in the maintenance of health. It is difficult to keep from becoming overly enthusiastic when talking or writing about physical fitness and its role in health. Historically, physical culture fads, like food fads, have been offered to the public as cure-alls. I hope that, as we have discussed so many problems involved in health, that you will realize, and I can remember, that life is a very complex experience. There are hazards all along the way from many different things. Ben Franklin had a simple solution to a complex problem—"Early to bed, early to rise, Makes a man healthy, wealthy and wise." Ah, if it were only so, or if an exercise program could solve all our health risks, money problems, and lack of understanding, would it not be a wonderful solution? Active participation in a physical fitness program does not offer a cure-all for the problems of health maintenance. There is no evidence to imply that the malignant diseases involve persons who are physically fit any less than the inactive portion of our population. However, there is mounting evidence to show that the physically active suffer fewer cardiovascular illnesses than the sedentary. I believe we can come up with the evidence and present it in such a way that physical fitness will be acceptable as a true form of life insurance. I suspect that the amount of activity that will be required to offer protection to the heart and vessels will be such that it can be done in a reasonable amount of time and entail little or no financial cost.

Let us review some of the reports of benefit from physical fitness as they now exist in the medical literature. I am combining the benefits from many different articles in the list below. The format of the list is borrowed from Dr. Samuel Fox III. Dr. Fox has contributed a great deal to the medical literature in the area of physical fitness and prevention of coronary heart disease.

PHYSICAL FITNESS MAY

INCREASE:	DECREASE:
cardiac stroke volume	the heart rate
coronary collateral vascularization	myocardial irritability
myocardial efficiency	total body fat
size of blood vessels, including coronaries	serum triglycerides
calcium content of bone structure	serum cholesterol
red cell mass to blood volume ratio	platelet stickiness
tolerance to emotional stress	heart size
arterial oxygen content	blood pressure
efficiency of the peripheral blood return	peripheral vascular resistance
zest for living	nervous reflexes
diastolic portion of pulse cycle	reaction time
the ability to work	constipation
sexual ability—libido	gastric secretions
the efficiency of capillaries and arteries	psychological depressions

oxygen consumption	varicose veins
chest expansion	body calcium loss
total body muscle	rate of development of degenerative joint disease
renal plasma flow	premature ventricular contractions

The above list makes it clear that physical conditioning is good for many things. Because of my interest in this subject over the past several years, I have reviewed many books and medical articles in reference to the effects of exercise. Virtually every physiologist who studies the effect of exercise points to the dramatic reduction in resting pulse rate. The resting pulse of 65 or less and the ability of the pulse to return to a rate of 100 or less within 10 minutes of severe exercise are the most generally accepted medical signs of physical fitness. This represents the medical definition of "being in shape."

Why, then, with this medical evidence of the benefits of exercise, has the medical profession been so slow to prescribe exercise to the public? The answer is simple. Certain people have diseases that contraindicate physical fitness programs. Several lists of such diseases and their degree of contraindication have been published. One was published by the American Medical Association in 1971. Another list, since modified, appeared in *The Journal of Preventive Medicine* in March 1972. It is presented in Chart number XXXIV in the Appendix. It is directed primarily to physicians who are examining patients for exercise tolerance. It will therefore appear technical. However, if you recognize in this list disorders that involve you, you can understand why your physician will advise you against exercise programs. In addition, it is difficult to identify the person who has only slightly more than marginal coronary blood flow. The evidence for this is clearly seen in the sudden death data. Remember that, in the Baltimore series of victims of sudden death, no less than 92 per cent of these persons had seen their physician within the last month. Therefore, when a physician tells a patient to embark on a physical fitness program and assures him that he is capable of participation, he assumes more than a little responsibility. He is aware of the limitations that may surround the patient with marginal coronary circulation, and he is also aware that the additional stress of exercise may precipitate a sudden death situation. We have spent considerable time in this text explaining the mechanism by which this can occur. As physicians we must therefore ask for your participation and your help in avoiding this situation. Again I would like to refer to my conversation with Dr. William Kannel, director of the Framingham project. He clearly stated that his greatest concern in terms of public programs for physical fitness would be that we would cover our streets with dead joggers. Everyone realizes that it is our purpose in advocating physical fitness to reduce these stress deaths! It is our desire to reduce this risk and to improve the quality and quantity of life. Therefore, the person participating in such a program must not start at a pace too vigorous for him and he must build up the pace of physical exercise over a relatively long period of time. *You* are the best person in the world to know when *you* are short of breath. *You* are the best person in the world to know when *you* are tired. *You* are the best person in the world to know when your endurance has been stressed to a significant degree. It is at this point that *you* must refrain from being competitive. *You* must accept your physical limitations. *You* must accept the importance of patience in achieving this important goal.

The above statements are made with all the force I can command in order to elicit your honest evaluation of your own ability. It is not my desire to deter you from starting a physical fitness program. I agree with the statements that have been attributed to several different authors that go something like this: Every person who wishes to enter a physical fitness program should have a physical checkup. But in light of our national epidemic of myocardial infarction, it may be even more important that people have a physical examination to see if they are capable of, or if it is reasonably safe for them to, remain sedentary. In other words, participating in an active program may have a risk, but not participating in some type of physical activity may have a risk that is even higher.

Like medicine, exercise should be prescribed. However, in most instances those who cannot tolerate exercise can be identified, and the prescription for the rest of the population can be a more general one. The implication is that exercise is a potent health tool, that, if used improperly, can be fatal. Our goal in this portion of the text is to see to it that you are on a safe, properly prescribed, exercise program. The first step in that prescription is to see to it that you do not have the contraindications to exercise as listed in our previous table. Once that hurdle is cleared, we can proceed to more specific advice.

If you are familiar with Dr. Kenneth Cooper's *Aerobics* and if you have been following his point system for developing physical fitness, we certainly wish you to continue to do so. Dr. Cooper has had extensive experience in physically conditioning men in the Air Force and has developed a very sensible physical fitness program. He has done a great deal to get Americans out of their soft chairs and into physically active programs.

I have so much appreciation of Dr. Cooper's work that I hesitate to be critical in any way. However, I advance one criticism. Under the Cooper system, a given distance in a given time is worth a certain number of points, and a weekly total of points is suggested. This is fine for a relatively uniform population such as the Air Force. It is less practical in a cross-section of the total population. The chubby sedentary female will stress herself infinitely more than the reasonably well-conditioned young or even middle-aged male to achieve the same point total.

A system I offer is quite simple. Since it is directed to all age groups and to all people in any state of physical condition, providing they pass the contraindication list and a stress EKG, we believe it safe. This system is based primarily on pulse rate. It is our belief that the muscle that needs the most tender loving care and at the same time needs to be built up to a fine edge of efficiency is the heart muscle. The only way this can be done is to exercise it. You cannot expect to build up your arm muscles unless you lift weights. You cannot expect to build up the leg muscles unless they are used. The same is true of the heart. The only way you can improve its efficiency and increase its stroke volume and minute volume is to stimulate it intermittently. I have repeatedly referred to your resting pulse. This is the starting place. If your resting pulse is 70 or below at the beginning of the program, you are in better condition than some of your neighbors. If your resting pulse is 80, you have a long way to go. If it is above that, you will need to proceed with caution. Even if your pulse rate is below 70, don't feel too smug. It may be that your pulse will not return to its normal rate following exercise as fast as it should. See Chart XXI. In order to stress your heart and make it strong, you must produce tachycardia. We have gone to great lengths to explain why too much tachycardia is a dangerous phenomenon. At this point we wish to introduce the term, "maximum heart rate." This is defined as that rate which is all the heart can tolerate, and this rate cannot be endured for prolonged periods of time. It must not be permitted to last more than 30 minutes, or medical help will most certainly be required. The maximum heart rate varies with age. When one is starting the physical fitness program one should consider the maximum heart rate to equal 220 minus your age in years. As the program proceeds and the heart becomes trained to shorten its systolic contraction time, the maximum heart rate may be calculated on the basis of 210 minus your age/2. Chart XXII shows the maximum heart rate as determined by Dr. S. Fox's formula, and we have added a second curve showing 70 per cent of that maximum heart rate. The second curve is introduced because a number of authors, particularly Dr. Raab of Vermont, have emphasized that, in order to acquire a conditioning effect on the heart, the exercise stress must produce a tachycardia equivalent to at least 70 per cent of the maximum heart rate. That area between these lines at your age is the range of heart rate necessary for conditioning. The basics of the conditioning program should be quite apparent. You will need to participate in some activity that will raise your pulse rate to at least 70 per cent of the maximum heart rate and hold it there for a given period of time. This period of time should be increased as conditioning improves. The following schedule is suggested. Week 1: 5 minutes. Week 2: 7 minutes. Week 3: 8 minutes. Weeks 4-5: 10 minutes. Weeks 6 through 12: 12 minutes. Weeks 13 through 20: 15 minutes. Thereafter, 30 minutes. It should be pointed out that a constant pace is not required to maintain an elevated pulse. Should you become quite short of breath or become uncomfortable from chest pain or undue fatigue, the pace can be reduced, the pulse can be checked, and the pace kept at a low rate until the pulse rate falls to the 70 per cent figure. The pace can then be increased as tolerated. If symptoms persist, it may be necessary to accept a walking pace only. You may find that walking alone will produce the necessary heart rate. This is particularly applicable to the jog-and-walk situation. Let us assume the following: A person with a resting pulse of 75 plans to start a walk-and-jog program; at the time he starts walking, his pulse will probably have increased to the mid 80's. He should walk rapidly or jog very slowly and check his pulse occasionally. When it reaches 110, we can assume that he has become prepared for more strenuous activity (this is the warm-up period) and at this point he will start to jog (not run) more vigorously. One minute after starting, the pulse rate should be checked, and at this point it should be at or above the 70 per cent of the maximum rate. Timekeeping begins at the point where the pulse reaches that rate. You now need five minutes of activity at this cardiac conditioning rate. If there is uncomfortable shortness of breath after the next minute of jogging, the pace may be slowed. Again, the pulse should be taken; if it is moving toward the maximum pulse rate, the pace should be reduced to a comfortable walk. If, on the other hand, it is just above the 70 per cent rate, the pace can be slowed for a short period and then a faster rate resumed.

In this manner, one's physical condition can self-regulate the amount of exercise and the pace. Some practical points need to be made at this time. First of all, do not try to count the pulse of your wrist. It is far easier to feel the heart pound on the anterior chest wall or palpate the larger and more active vessels in the neck. Feel directly back from the angle of the jaw, directing the fingers toward the midline and slightly downward and the pulse should be readily palpable. A wrist watch with a second hand or stop watch will be needed to time the pulse. With a little practice, a five-second count will be adequate to give a reasonably good reading of the pulse rate, although initially it may require ten seconds. During the time when the pulse is being taken, it will be necessary to slow to a walk, but it should not be necessary to come to a standstill. It is important that you not come to a standstill at any time until the pulse has returned to well under the 70-per cent level and preferably to a point approximately 20 beats per minute below the 70-per cent range. A number of authors have warned against too rapid deceleration, for it is during the period following exercise that the venous return to the heart is most altered and it is at this time that premature contractions or irregularities of the pulse occur. Dr. Cooper was very specific in his warning in this point. More recently Dr. Earl Beard reported to the 9th International Congress of Cardiology that some 11 per cent of executives with a mean age of 40 developed irregularity following exercise. This again implies that the time of greatest risk is the five to ten minutes following the exercise period. Activity of a reduced type must be maintained over this interval to permit the heart to adapt to the changing venous return.

It is important that you be especially careful to avoid those things that increase myocardial irritability in the post-exercise period. Do not shower with either hot or cold water until the pulse rate is at or within 15 beats of pre-exercise levels. Avoid cold or hot drinks, including alcohol or coffee, for at least an hour after exercise. Rapid changes in the environmental temperature are most important; steam rooms and air conditioning should be avoided. Such drugs as nicotine and caffeine may increase the post-exercise risk.

I have implied that you will adopt a walk-and-jog program for exercise. This is not necessarily true. Any activity that can increase the pulse rate as indicated can serve as a conditioning exercise for the heart. Swimming, bicycling, or even walking may be perfectly adequate to stimulate the heart rate in the desired manner. However, as conditioning improves, it will be necessary to increase the activity in order to raise the pulse rate to the desired level. One of my physician colleagues, who is in very excellent condition, can no longer force his pulse rate up to 150 by running at the customary pace for a 3-mile run. He requires an initial sprint, then can reduce his pace to a more conventional one geared for distance. One publication suggests that sexual activity may be adequate for physical conditioning. Theoretically, this seems feasible, for the pulse rate must increase with sexual endeavors. However, I seriously doubt that it would be convenient to check the pulse under such circumstances! It would also require that this level of activity be maintained for 30 minutes and that, as conditioning improved, the duration and intensity be increased. It has also been stated that weight can be lost as a result of sexual exercise; however, I would emphasize that running at the rate of 7 miles per hour burns approximately 150 calories per mile. In fact, this is a maximum reported calorie usage. Perhaps sexual activity is as efficient as running when it comes to burning calories; there are no scientific experiments to confirm or deny this. However, since most forms of exercise are relatively inefficient ways of reducing weight, it would seem that, to obtain dramatic changes in weight reduction from sexual activity, it would need to be substituted for the evening meal.

The frequency with which one carries out the exercise program is important. The figures, as we have listed them, are based on a five-day week. If one wishes to increase the amount of time each day as training progresses, the number of days may be reduced. We all have days that lend themselves less favorably to the addition of extracurricular activities. It is suggested that one not exercise seven days a week, but that the week be broken up, with a day off sometime during the middle of the week. A 4-5 day exercise week is suggested as ideal. After conditioning is attained, one can maintain, but not improve, conditioning with 30-40 minutes three times per week.

Such sports as weightlifting and calisthenics can be used in the training program for developing muscular balance and coordination. However, it is difficult to raise the pulse rate to an adequate level unless one participates in one of the more vigorous sports. One of the cardiology fellows at our hospital suggested to me that it might be possible for the heart to be trained without the use of physical exercise. He was suggesting a passive form of conditioning. Such a program would include either a steam bath or sauna to the point where the body temperature is elevated and the pulse rate goes up to 70 per cent of maximum range. This sounded like an exciting possibility, and we promptly tried it. I became extremely uncomfortable in both the sauna and steam room; even when the discomfort was such that it was virtually intolerable, my pulse could not be raised above 110 and this was still below 70 per cent of maximum pulse rate. However, my physical condition was reasonably good at this time. My colleague had the same experience. Therefore, while passive cardiac exercise is intriguing, it cannot be recommended. Since this experience I have learned from Dr. Fox that this may be a dangerous experiment, especially for the poorly conditioned person. Steam and sauna baths are now prevalent in apartment houses and health clubs. The combination of poor physical condition, heat, and humidity may be a fatal one.

You will note that our progressive exercise plan does not include any given distances, whether in running, swimming, or jogging. Early in the course of training, it is best that the trainee not compete with others or with the clock. After the initial 12-week period has been completed, there are certainly advantages in keeping records of one's progress. I know of no better way than following Dr. Cooper's 12-minute exercise fitness test. This requires the trainee to run, walk, or crawl continuously for 12 minutes and record the distance traversed. One of the real pleasures of physical fitness training is the progressive improvement that one can observe as the months go by. I suggest that, after this initial 12-week period, you record the distance you can travel in 12 minutes, or during your routine 30-minute period. Keep a record on the calendar each time you exercise and record the performance accomplished. This does not mean that you should try every day to better the performance of the day before. There is no question that you will find periods in which you will do well and other times in which you perform at less than your peak. As one conditions oneself, there will be periods in which the performance reaches a plateau; then, unexpectedly, it will improve again. If you continue the program for a period of one year, you will be truly amazed at the improvement in your performance.

The weather will certainly be a prime factor in your performance. This is especially true if you are participating in a walk-jog-run program. Walk-jog-run programs are virtually the only ones that can be participated in on a year-round basis. Others such as swimming can be participated in all year if special facilities are available. The extremes of temperature in which one should exercise are dependent upon the area of the country in which one lives. It also depends a great deal upon how well adjusted you are to the climate at this particular moment. It would be foolish to start a running program in 100-degree weather if you are not well acclimatized. It would also be discouraging to start a program in zero weather unless you are accustomed to this type of climate. If one does start or perform under adverse conditions, checking the pulse is very important, for in this way you let the heart rate tell you how all stresses are being absorbed. Even though I am reasonably well conditioned, I find running outdoors difficult if the temperature is over 95°. At the other extreme, with warm clothing one can run outdoors at virtually any temperature unless the wind is blowing. I should add that a snow-packed surface is ideal for running. I am inclined to move indoors if the temperature is under 20 or 30° if there is a wind blowing. When the temperature becomes prohibitive outdoors, some form of indoor exercise is needed. The mode of exercise used will depend a great deal on the facilities available. Basketball or swimming are excellent, provided a gym or indoor pool is available. My personal solution to this problem was the purchase of a treadmill. The treadmill is slightly inclined. It is heavy enough to be stable and is powered only by the runner. I personally find 30 minutes on this exhausting. There is no difficulty in producing an adequate tachycardia. In terms of time utilization, this beats all other forms of exercise. Whenever I use it, I try to time its usage so I can watch the news on television at the same time. This prevents the treadmilling experience from being too boring. By this method you can simultaneously accomplish physical fitness and keep abreast of the news. One of my cardiology friends has an indoor stationary bicycle. This accomplishes the same purpose; he can watch the news and exercise at the same time. I do not use the treadmill routinely because I do not enjoy it. Running outdoors is much more pleasant, though less efficient. Indoor stationary running is another means by which the limitations of the weather can be avoided. It is similar to stationary bicycling or treadmill exercise. Stationary running may be more economical in that it requires no outlay of money for equipment. I find it extremely hard to do. One of my physician friends has an indoor walking track in his basement. It goes behind the furnace, around a ping pong table, and back. He does this very religiously on days he cannot tolerate outdoor conditions.

As I have implied, there are many ways of exercising. It can be modified to meet the prevailing weather conditions and one's personal tastes. However, even if one starts with a low-intensity exercise such as walking or playing golf, and conditioning improves, one will find himself forced into the cross-country skiing, jog-and-run, bicycling, or swim-type programs, for these are the forms of exercise vigorous enough to force the pulse rate into the training range. It should be mentioned that exercise programs can be mixed. On some occasions, even in nice weather, I may use the treadmill just to break the routine. Swimming on one exercise day each week is also a good break in the running routine.

The type of clothing worn depends a great deal upon

the weather. In cold weather some type of warm clothing is required. A classic gray sweatshirt and trousers are acceptable. If it is cold and a wind is blowing, it may be necessary to wear additional clothing beneath the sweat suit. Gloves or mittens are necessary even in cool weather. Cold hands are very annoying; it seems that, after a short period of running, one tends to feel warm all over, except for the hands. In hot weather it is important that heat from the body be permitted to escape. The nylon sweat suits that I see on some joggers are mentioned only to be condemned. They are sold with the claim of helping to lose weight. Certainly, they increase the body heat. This results in loss of water, which will be restored shortly after the exercise period. Hot weather running wear should be light-weight, loose-fitting track trunks with or without a T-shirt. In this way the body heat can be dissipated rapidly.

If you are just starting a walk-jog-run program, there is nothing more important than the type of footwear. Virtually everyone who participates in a jogging exercise program will eventually have some foot and leg problems. Most of these are minor; a good many can be prevented. If you have obvious mechanical problems as far as the legs and feet are concerned, maybe it is best that you derive your exercise from swimming or bicycling. Such problems include bowlegs, knockknees, flat feet, or an unusually high arch. For most people a cross-country running shoe which has an arch support and thick soft sole is the most satisfactory to wear. Don't get discouraged when there is considerable foot and leg soreness. Slow down the pace of outdoor activity and use the swimming pool more. The standard white wool and nylon sock is very satisfactory, as is any comfortable sock that is absorbent. If you are going to be committed to a training program that will be continued indefinitely, there is no reason why you shouldn't equip yourself in the best manner possible.

What Physical Fitness Will Not Do

I have tried to project my enthusiasm for a physical fitness program. It is the one thing everyone can do that will improve not only his physical fitness, but also his self-esteem. If improvement of one's self-esteem were the only product of a physical fitness program, it would still be worthwhile. However, improvement seems to go well beyond this. Exercise programs involve physiological processes of the anti-aging type. If you will recall, we made a similar statement in the section dealing with arteriosclerosis. We do not wish to imply that exercise programs specifically decrease the amount of atherosclerosis. This has not been proven and should be classed as one of the things exercise will not do. However, I must admit some developing evidence has a strong implication that one of the long term effects of exercise, by reducing triglycerides, will protect against atherosclerosis. Arteriosclerotic processes seem to be more closely related to diet and hereditary metabolic processes than to any form of physical fitness.

However, the aging process is slowed by maintaining excellent blood flow to all vital organs. By decreasing the amount of atherosclerosis, adequate blood flow to vital organs is accomplished by maintaining vessels of normal caliber to these organs. One can also increase the blood flow to a given area by exercise. The mechanism by which this occurs is somewhat different. Exercise reduces the peripheral resistance and thus increases blood flow. Exercise programs reduce aging primarily of the muscles and joints and that very important muscle, the heart. It has also been shown that exercise programs tend to increase the renal blood flow, extremely important in the maintenance of normal life in the late years.

Despite the above paragraph, we listed on page 212 "long-term vigorous exercise programs" as an acceptable means of lowering cholesterol. Thirty minutes of vigorous exercise (7.5 cal/min) four or five times per week will not qualify. A study done at the University of Illinois has shown that a program of 45 minutes per day 5 days per week at an intensity of 10-12 calories per minute can lower cholesterol, and Dr. Bassler, our marathon enthusiast, feels that marathoners can eat anything. He gives no laboratory data, but the marathoner is trained at levels well above those required to lower cholesterol. Most people cannot or will not, train to this degree. As for us, we cannot abandon the low fat diet. We will follow Dr. Irving Page's famous advice to those wishing to avoid heart attacks: "Get off your fatty acids and run!"

It is a well-known fact that some trained athletes have died of myocardial infarction. Athletic skill in itself is no guarantee against this disorder. This is especially true if the given individual comes from a family with a high incidence of arteriosclerosis or if the individual himself has other high risk factors, such as elevated blood pressure, anomalies of the coronary vessels, or addiction to smoking. Physical training can lessen the effect of other risks, but it cannot negate them. Athletes may develop special skills and still be poorly conditioned by our cardiac criteria.

Exercise programs should not be used primarily for weight control. You will notice on our chart of contraindications for exercise programs that one indication for additional or specific medical supervision is marked obesity. Anyone who is grossly overweight, should reduce by a strict diet prior to embarking on an exercise program. While the program itself will help in the control of obesity, it is not nearly as efficient as avoiding the intake of food. It seems that anyone weighing over 200 pounds may develop orthopedic problems to the point where running programs are impractical. Such persons will need to swim or bicycle. We have previously stated that one burns approximately 150 calories while running a mile at the rate of 7 miles per hour. This 150 calories is approximately equivalent to one martini. However, if one substitutes a mile run for that one martini, there is a net reduction of 300 calories. If one uses exercise in this way, it can have a very significant effect on weight problems. I should also add that there is every reason to believe that a one- or two-mile run is as relaxing as, and perhaps more so, than one or two martinis. However, if one were trying to substitute exercise for 1000 calories of intake, one would need to run 6.6 miles, and most people would find that a difficult chore. It may surprise you to find that, after a year of our program, a six- or seven-mile run is not at all impossible—in fact, it is quite easy. It is obvious that exercise can serve as an aid in the control of obesity, but unfortunately weight reduction must still be primarily a diet program. Exercise may complement the weight-reduction program in another way. It is a common experience to lose weight promptly on a diet—then in a few weeks, on the same diet, to note little change. Part of this paradox is a change in metabolic rate; after the initial weight loss, the metabolic rate lowers and weight loss is more difficult. When exercise is added to the diet, this lowering of the metabolic rate does not occur and the loss is more encouraging. In this way exercise is worth more than the calories specifically burned. See Chart XXXV in the Appendix.

There are a number of other things that physical fitness will not do for you. As I have mentioned before, it will not protect you from cancer. Neither does it protect you from accidents or homicide. It will not earn your daily bread or pay your taxes; however, it will give you a much more vigorous outlook on life. You will enjoy an improved self-image, and the evidence from many sources suggests that you will live a longer and more healthy life if you remain active. To paraphrase Dr. Samuel Fox III again, exercise programs may add years to your life and will certainly add life to your years.

XII. Decades of Disaster or Delight

Ages 45-54 and 55-64

For the first time we shall consider two decades together. This is done to avoid repetition. The leading killers are now well established; only the numbers they kill in each decade will change. These numbers can be clearly derived from Charts XXIII and XXIV.

The general statistical information for these decades includes the fact that the age group between 45 and 54 contains 22,538,000 people. Therefore, to obtain the approximate actual number of deaths per given entry, multiply the entry number by 225.4. In the age group 55-64 there were 17,572,000 people; therefore, to obtain the actual number of deaths per given entry multiply the number on the chart by 175.7. All entries in our mortality tables are showing an increase with increasing age. The one exception to this is homicide, and here the trends starts down at age 34. The decreasing death rate from accidents continues through age 45 and 54, but turns upward in the 55-to-64 age group. The death rates from malignancy and major cardiovascular renal diseases continue to show tremendous increases; however, they now appear to be doubling with each decade rather than tripling, as we noted previously. Diabetes with a threefold increase and pulmonary emphysema with a nearly fourfold increase in death rate show the greatest change percentagewise between our two decades of interest.

Because of the continued marked preponderance of major cardiovascular renal disease as a cause of death, a breakdown of the components of the major entity is again offered.

Cardiac Disease	45-54	55-64
Rheumatic heart disease	12.2	21.8
Arteriosclerotic heart disease and coronary heart disease	211.8	594.0
Hypertensive heart disease	16.4	42.8
Other heart disease	11.7	28.8
Vascular Disease		
CNS (strokes)	43.5	130.9
Generalized arteriosclerosis	1.3	8.3
Peripheral manifestations and hypertension	3.8	7.0
Other general vascular disease	11.3	30.4

This chart is similar to the data we presented for the last decade; however, the numbers grow continuously larger. The magnitude of the coronary heart disease problem remains apparent; when we review the total statistics for all age groups over the past ten years, we find that the incidence of coronary heart disease and its complications has shown a slow but steady increase. The mortality rate of 300 per 100,000 has increased to 316.3 per 100,000 in the past ten years. This has taken place during the period when all forms of heart disease are showing a slight but definite decrease in mortality rate. This decrease in mortality has been particularly evident in hypertensive heart disease, where the rate has fallen from 42.7 per 100,000 in 1958 to 25.3 in 1967. The later data are not age-corrected, but apply to all age groups in the indicated years.

The Respiratory System

It now seems fitting to review some of the features of lung anatomy and physiology that are important to your health. In speaking of the respiratory system, it is natural to think primarily of the lungs. They are the major organ involved, but other structures are equally important. These include the nasal cavity, the larynx, the trachea, the major bronchi, the small bronchi, the diaphragm, and the chest wall. If any of these ancillary areas are compromised, the lungs will be seriously handicapped. It is the role of the lungs to serve as the area of gas exchange between the body and the outside atmosphere. In order to do this effectively, outside oxygen containing air must be drawn into the lungs. The exchange takes place at the cell membrane level, and the expired gas is replaced by air containing a larger percentage of oxygen.

The upper respiratory tract consists of the area from the tip of the nose to the smallest subdivision of the bronchus and serves as the passageway for the exchanged air; it also acts as an air-conditioning system that controls the temperature and humidity of the air entering the lung itself. In addition to this control system, the upper respiratory tract has another extremely important function. This deals with the removal of the foreign material breathed into the airway. The hair in the nose serves first as a coarse filter that removes large particles drawn into the airway on inspiration. The trachea and bronchi are lined with mucus-secreting glands and cells. A thin layer of mucus formed by these glands serves as an excellent trap for debris that is drawn into the airway. In addition to this, the mucus is driven away from the lung by a remarkably efficient ciliary system. The cilia are tiny hairlike projections extending out from the cells of the bronchus. They whip or drive the mucus as a blanket back toward the nose and throat. In this way, the particulate foreign material that enters the airway is trapped and very efficiently returned to the nose and throat, where it may be coughed out or swallowed. In these days of air pollution, this cleansing system of the respiratory tract is of the utmost importance; damage to this apparatus is dangerous to your health.

The trachea is a midline structure approximately an inch in diameter. It divides into major bronchi, one to the right and one to the left lung. Each of these major bronchi divide many times into smaller bronchi until they reach a point where the lining epithelial cells of the bronchus change and are no longer mucus-secreting and cilia-containing. At this point we refer to the structure as a terminal bronchiole, and from here on there is direct communication from this structure and the outpouching sacs, the alveoli. The size of the lung is proportional to the size of the patient, particularly his height. We are told that in the average man there are some 35,000 terminal bronchioles and that these communicate with 300,000,000 alveoli. To further emphasize the great surface area of the lung that results from this arrangement, it has been demonstrated that the average surface area of one lung, if it could be stretched out into a single plane, would be about 900 square feet. Since each lung contains approximately one pint of blood at any given moment, you can see how thin a layer of the blood is spread over this large surface. It is in the alveolus that the surface of the lung and the surface of the blood-containing capillary are intimately related, and here gas exchange takes place.

The pulmonary arterial system, as it leaves the heart, follows the course of the bronchial tree. The branches of the pulmonary arteries tend to parallel those of the bronchus. The pulmonary arteries, like arteries described elsewhere, have a muscular layer and are capable of contracting and dilating. However, by the time the arteries reach the level of the terminal bronchioles, they lose their continuous muscle coat and become a thinner structure. Shortly after this they break into the capillary network that surrounds and is intimately related to the alveolus.

Just as the heart muscle must have its own blood supply, the lung also must have a source of systemic arterial blood. The blood supply to the lungs arises either directly from the aorta or from one of its branches. They supply the bronchial walls as far as the terminal bronchioles and also act as a source of oxygen for the nerves and lymphatic structures that also must exist in the tissue between the blood vessel coming from the heart and the air sacs. The blood supply to the lung itself is quite rich and apparently more than adequate, since we know of no death or disease that results from obstruction of one or more of these arteries. Some theories regarding the origin of emphysema involve the bronchial arteries, but these are unproven and not generally accepted.

Physicians have many ways of examining the respiratory tract. These vary from such simple things as watching the patient breathe or listening to the breath sounds with a stethoscope to the more complicated studies that involve analysis of venous or arterial blood for its oxygen and carbon dioxide content. Direct visualization of the trachea and bronchi can be done through a long slender tube, a bronchoscope. Other anatomical details are visualized through chest X-rays and chest fluoroscopy; the arteries can be visualized by injecting opaque material into the pulmonary artery itself or into the bronchial arteries through the aorta. Functional studies of the lung can also vary in their degree of complexity. In a sense, listening to the breath sounds is both a physiological and anatomical examination of the lungs. It is also true that we gain a certain amount of physiological information from chest films and chest fluoroscopy. At fluoroscopy, we can see the action of the diaphragm and may find a clue to the fact that one lung is not aerating as well as the other. We can also identify a diaphragm that is not functioning properly. If a diaphragm is not moving, lung efficiency is reduced by about 25 per cent. However, most of the pulmonary function studies are carried out in the laboratory, where volumes of air can be measured accurately. Even in a laboratory where many tests are available, these tend to be of varying complexity. One of the most valuable tests and a relatively simple one to do is that of vital capacity. This is simply a measure of the amount of air that can be expelled from the airway following full inspiration. In our discussions of preventing myocardial infarction, we suggested that a better than normal vital capacity seemed to offer protection against myocardial infarction. These data were derived from the Framingham study. They used 2300 cc maximum expiration for a female and 3000 cc maximum expiration for a male as a dividing line between normal and below normal. Most pulmonary physiologists would not be so lenient with their values, for a normal value varies with the age and height of the patient. Pulmonary function laboratories therefore use charts to plot patients' ages and heights against given values and a range of normal. Thus, they can be more specific and more individualized in the results of function studies. A vital capacity of 3000 cc would seem to be adequate for most males; however, if the male were tall and young, 3000 cc might actually represent a low vital capacity. Certainly one of the most important findings in lung function is a decreasing vital capacity. If one has serial measurements over the years and finds that the vital capacity is falling at a rate faster than would be anticipated with age, we have an important sign of pulmonary disease. This is also a warning that myocardial infarction may be impending. There are many variations on the theme of vital capacity function. For instance, the measurement of the amount of air that can be forced out by rapid expiration in one second has become a popular test. One crude lung function test on this same general order can be performed by anyone. A lighted match held to full arm's length should be easily extinguished with one rapid expiratory puff. If this cannot be done, the patient has reduced lung function. Since we did not define the type of match or the arm length, you can see why we called the test crude.

There are many other measurements the physiology laboratory can do with accuracy. These include the determinations of the total lung volume, maximum inspiratory volume, and residual lung volume. These terms should not be frightening; maximum inspiratory volume is just that, it is the number of cubic centimeters of air that can be drawn in on maximum inspiration. Vital capacity has already been defined as forced expiration following maximum inspiration. The residual volume in the lung is that which remains after maximum expiration. Total lung volume is vital capacity plus residual lung volume. It is also possible and helpful on occasion to measure the airway resistance.

The most discouraging aspect of evaluating lung disease is related to nature's generosity. Even when a portion of lung is destroyed, there is enough remaining lung tissue adequately to oxygenate all of the blood being sent to it by the heart. Since the patient will have no symptoms, he will not see his physician. Even if he saw his physician and many of the tests were done, the changes from the normal might still be relatively minor compared to the seriousness of the disease process that is developing. Even if some of the tests showed abnormality, it would then be a problem to localize the portion of the lung involved or to determine whether the lung as a whole was diffusely diseased. However, most of us feel we can cope with that problem. The greater problem is persuading patients who feel normal to have a simple test such as that for vital capacity. If findings are abnormal and if the patient is feeling well, it may be equally difficult to persuade him to follow any therapeutic regime. You will note that I have said very little about exercise tolerance tests for lung function. Exercise performance is certainly dependent upon an efficient gas exchange system. Again, because of its rather extensive reserve, the lung is not usually the limiting factor in exercise. The limiting factor is the heart. Therefore, unless there is lung disease, exercise tolerance or intolerance, as the case may be, is usually a cardiac problem rather than a pulmonary one. Exercise tolerance tests can be used in patients with extensive lung disease in an attempt to evaluate the limitations that this lung disease produces. It has even been used as a part of therapy for patients with chronic lung disease.

Diseases of the Lung

Not many years ago, the phrase "lung disease" immediately brought thoughts of tuberculosis. Tuberculosis has not been totally eradicated. In our year of 1967, 6351 people died of tuberculosis of the respiratory tract. However, this represents a dramatic drop from the figures of previous decades. We are now less concerned about tuberculosis than we are about such diseases as emphysema and cancer of the lung, the incidence of which is rapidly increasing. One of the great improvements of medicine in the last 50 years has been the decreasing incidence of tuberculosis. Pediatric wards no longer house the numerous pathetic cases of tuberculous meningitis that were present even 25 years ago. At that time, even adults had a far greater incidence of tuberculosis than we now encounter. There were separate tuberculosis hospitals in virtually every city, and one of the real risks of being a young medical student on the medical wards was that of exposure to tuberculosis. Many a young physician contracted the disease as a result of examining infective patients. The decreased incidence of tuberculosis is a reflection of improved medical treatment and our generally improved standard of living. The public health experts have played a big role in case-finding and in follow-up care. Other areas of the world are not so fortunate; because Americans make extended visits outside of the United States, I am certain that tuberculosis will never completely disappear from this country.

The most common disease of the respiratory system that has mortality significance is pneumonia. Antibiotics have resulted in a very high rate of cure of this disease. We should, in general, speak of infectious disease of the respiratory tract. If we have a runny nose, general aches and pains, and no fever, we call it a cold. If there is an associated sore throat, with hoarseness of the voice, this is laryngitis. If there is an associated productive cough, again with no fever, this is bronchitis. When the infectious process extends to the alveolus, it has spread to a point where the protective mechanism of the cilia and mucus can no longer help in defense. Drainage is poor, fever will be present, and the result is pneumonia. Some pneumonias are not bacterial. Since these may be caused by viruses or a variety of organisms, the etiology of pneumonia must be determined by culture or by clinical and X ray characteristics.

Bacteria can reach the alveolus by either of two routes. The usual route is through the air passages, as described above. The other route by which bacteria can reach the alveolus is through transport by the bloodstream. This implies an infectious process elsewhere in the body, an invasion of the bloodstream, and entrapment or filtering out of these organisms by the lung. This generally results in a more serious form of pneumonia than those that enter through the airways. Most airway pneumonias are caused by the pneumococcus organism, while the organisms that produce pneumonia of the blood-borne type can be various, depending upon the infectious process. One of the most common blood-borne types of pneumonia is caused by the staphylococcus, which can be secondary to such a simple thing as a pimple or boil. Blood-borne types of pneumonia are much less common than the airborne varieties. At the same time, we are thankful that it was the lung that filtered this organism and trapped it in preference to throwing it back into the circulation, where it might have gone to the brain.

In 1967 the vital statistics book lists pneumonia, except pneumonia of the newborn, as taking 55,470 lives. If we add influenza and pneumonia of the newborn, we arrive at a figure of well over 60,000 deaths, and this becomes a very significant number. In these days of high cure rates with antibiotics, this seems an unusual and unnecessarily high number. I am sure that this number will always remain high, for deaths from pneumonia are too often the result of a complication. To the elderly patient who has had a stroke, who has had a hip fracture pinned, or who is disabled from some other cause, pneumonia is the final blow. Certainly, as one looks at the incidence of death from pneumonia according to decade of life, it is quite apparent that the rate increases rapidly after the age of 75. Death from pneumonia in the productive middle years of life does occur, but its incidence is relatively low. Respiratory infections will always be with us. From a preventive standpoint it is well to remember that, by coughing, the droplets of a disease can be spread to those who are not involved. Virtually all forms of upper respiratory infections are therefore communicable diseases. Your resistance is very important.

Chronic Obstructive Pulmonary Disease

The term "chronic obstructive pulmonary disease" includes two entities. One is chronic bronchitis, the other pulmonary emphysema. These disorders are discussed together because they share many similarities and usually occur together. Some authors feel that pulmonary emphysema is the end product of chronic bronchitis. In other words, it is the same disease in a more advanced form. I personally like that theory, although I must admit that there are features of pulmonary emphysema that are difficult to explain on this basis.

Chronic bronchitis is basically defined as the production of too much mucus in the bronchial tree. There may or may not be superimposed infection. When there is, this implies a second process, which probably should be referred to as an acute bronchitis superimposed on a chronic bronchitis. From the standpoint of the patient, chronic bronchitis is a nagging, irritating productive cough. If there is no sputum, interrogation of the patient usually reveals the fact that sputum is swallowed rather than expectorated. Chronic bronchitis results in moderate shortness of breath since the mucus in the airway decreases its caliber, especially that of the smaller airways as the major bronchi divide. The vital capacity is reduced.

When radiographic studies of the bronchi are performed in patients with chronic bronchitis, it is very evident that there is hypertrophy of the mucus-secreting glands and that the bronchi are somewhat larger and not as elastic as those in the normal patient. Simple chronic bronchitis is listed as the cause of death of 5306 patients in 1967. As a contributing factor to such other disease as pulmonary emphysema, heart failure, and pneumonia, the number would be much greater. Chronic bronchitis is a relatively common disease, produces considerable morbidity, and contributes to mortality primarily through other diseases. The complication of bronchitis is nowhere more evident than in the postoperative patient. Post operative lung complications occur ten times as often in the patient with bronchitis as in the patient with healthy lungs. Part of the routine preparation for elective surgery now includes lung cleansing to reduce postoperative complications. This lack of lung preparation increases the risk in emergency surgery unless the lungs are healthy.

Chronic bronchitis can vary a great deal in severity. This may be nothing more than an annoying morning cough; otherwise, the symptoms can be so exaggerated that clinically it is identical to pulmonary emphysema. It is at this point that a differential diagnosis between the two is attempted, for if the disease is basically chronic bronchitis, therapeutic regimes can bring about improvement. The difficulties in distinguishing between some forms of chronic bronchitis and pulmonary emphysema have resulted in the term "chronic obstructive pulmonary disease." This descriptive term includes both pathological processes.

For obvious reasons, pulmonary emphysema has been intensively investigated in the past 15 years. In 1950 approximately 3000 people in the United States died from pulmonary emphysema. In 1967 our vital statistics data indicate that 20,875 deaths were specifically attributed to pulmonary emphysema. This increase in the death rate has occurred primarily in the cities. In New York City the death rate from pulmonary emphysema has increased tenfold in ten years. The term emphysema implies destruction of the alveoli. When this occurs, therapy is of little or no value. However, if chronic bronchitis is associated with the emphysema, it may be that clearing the mucus from the tracheal bronchial tree may improve the patient's pulmonary function.

The mechanism of producing pulmonary emphysema may follow one of two routes. The most common and generally accepted theory is that the increased mucus production of the tracheal bronchial tree results in more fluid retention in the lung than it can tolerate. It is well known that the bronchi dilate with inspiration and contract with expiration. Therefore, as tenacious bits of mucus extend further down the bronchial tree, it is evident that a point is reached when air can get in and cannot escape. The results are the overinflation and eventual rupture of alveoli. This mechanism has been well documented in other disorders, and there seems to be little question that it is one of the predominant means of destroying alveoli. The other possible mechanism assumes that the bronchial arteries that nourish the bronchi are either small or are subject to chronic spastic effects and that as a result the distal bronchi and alveoli become damaged for want of oxygen. The latter theory is somewhat attractive when one looks at the vascular changes in the autopsy specimen, but these vascular changes could be secondary to the chronic intrinsic pulmonary disease. It is quite evident that, as the disease progresses, the airway resistance becomes greater. Initially, there is a reduced expiratory volume and therefore reduced vital capacity. As the disease progresses and the inspiratory volume is decreased, the air exchange is further depressed. The classic emphysematous lung is grossly overinflated.

Pulmonary emphysema is an insidious disease. We have already referred to the very great reserve of the lung. Patients who subsequently have advanced pulmonary emphysema usually date the onset of their illness to an infectious process or to the inhalation of a noxious gas; in fact, these are only precipitating factors that exhaust the last of the patient's pulmonary reserve. By the time symptoms become manifest to such a point that the patient seeks a physician's advice, the damage is extensive. It has been estimated that these patients lose from 1 to 2 per cent of their lung function each year. If the patient lives his life so that no physicial stress is required, it may be 20 to 25 years before symptoms develop. The effect of chronic obstructive pulmonary disease, especially emphysema, on the heart deserves some comment. As the alveoli over-inflate, the total gas capacity of the lung increases. The space readily available for the blood is decreased. This means increased peripheral vascular resistance in the lung bed. As a result, the pressure in the pulmonary artery rises, in many instances by a factor of three to four. An extra work load is placed on the right ventricle, which is not designed to carry the maximum pressure that is common to the left ventricle. At this point, the patient has two problems; not only does he have trouble getting adequate air in and out of his lungs to sustain even his sedentary life, but life now becomes complicated by an overworked and failing right ventricle. Those of you who think you may have a touch of bronchitis or a little emphysema should by all means see a physician. If he cannot impress upon you the importance of care, treatment, and prevention, you should then take the time to visit the chest wards of any large hospital. The veterans hospitals are filled with patients with chronic lung disease. There are very few situations that can put a man in a more trying position than to make him short of breath for 24 hours a day. Getting enough air to live becomes a full-time struggle. Mortality rates are only part of the story; disability is severe and may be present for many years before death. Since chronic obstructive pulmonary disease produces such great suffering and its mortality rate is rapidly increasing, the search to find a method for prevention has been intense.

Prevention of Chronic Obstructive Pulmonary Disease

A moderate amount of pulmonary emphysema will develop as an aging process. Therefore, any person who survives to the age of 80 or more can be expected to lose elasticity of pulmonary tissues that results in hyperaeration and some loss of alveolar function. However, this is a considerably different entity from the emphysema that we may see as early as age 40 or 50. This is mentioned only to indicate that research studies done on all age groups, particularly those late in life, will find a moderate degree of emphysema in virtually all elderly patients. Severe emphysema and severe chronic bronchitis are the enemies we are interested in identifying and preventing. A recent article by Dr. Oscar Auerbach in *The New England Journal of Medicine* gave a reported incidence of pulmonary emphysema. He reviewed entire lungs as examined at autopsy in 1831 patients. He found the incidence of severe pulmonary emphysema in the nonsmoking patient to be zero, but the incidence of advanced pulmonary emphysema to be 19.2 per cent in patients who smoked more than one pack of cigarettes per day. You will note that this is a cross-section study done on a relatively large number of patients who died from varying causes and not just from pulmonary diseases. Certainly the 19.2 per cent who had advanced pulmonary emphysema had symptoms. In the study, only the objective findings at autopsy and the historic data of cigarette consumption were used. This is not the first paper to incriminate cigarettes in the development of chronic obstructive pulmonary disease.

In the April 16, 1973 issue of *The Journal of the American Medical Association*, one group of physicians found 39 per cent incidence of emphysema in heavy smoking males who were victims of sudden death. These deaths were not caused directly by pulmonary disease, but the association of the pulmonary role in sudden death is clear. Similar changes were found in females to establish the dose relationship between smoking and emphysema. For the past several years the reports of the Surgeon General of the United States have stated that the evidence linking cigarettes to chronic obstructive disease was so strong that he was willing to state a cause-and-effect relationship between these entities. We do know that there are rare instances in which emphysema develops in a nonsmoker. One type of enzyme deficiency has been identified as a congenital defect.

These patients develop emphysema whether they smoke or not. It is also known that a small percentage of severe asthmatics may eventually develop emphysema to a significant degree, even in the absence of tobacco.

To make a more logical case, further relationships between smoking and chronic obstructive pulmonary disease are required. We need to review the effect of tobacco smoke on the respiratory tract. Cigarette smoke is a heterogenous mixture of gases, uncondensed vapors, and liquid particulate material. Several hundred different compounds have been isolated from tobacco and its smoke. These enter the oral cavity primarily as an aerosol of small particulate matter. The particles are drawn into the bronchi and, like particles of any type, they are in part captured by the mucus lining the bronchus. The mucus and cilia now attempt to remove them from the lung. However, it is here that the one great difference between particles brought into the lung by cigarette smoke and particles inhaled from conventional air pollution occurs. In addition to the particulate matter of the cigarette smoke, there are many gases and vapors, one of which is a very effective toxin to the cilia and serves to anesthetize them. Therefore, at the time when the particles should be beaten back from the lung, the cilia are put to sleep, the particles either enter the lung or are trapped in mucus that is present, and the first line of defense is shattered. Our second line of defense, that of secreting more mucus, is called upon. In response, an outpouring of mucus occurs. The mucus accumulates, and the cilia remain ineffective. The mucus can be removed voluntarily by the patient if he coughs. We have described the natural history and birth of the cigarette cough. This cough is an extremely important defense mechanism to the smoker. It has been shown to be quite effective in clearing the lung; unfortunately, it is of limited value during the sleeping hours or when it is voluntarily suppressed.

A number of unsuccessful tests have been done in an attempt to identify and possibly remove this ciliary toxic agent from cigarette smoke. Filters are ineffective. They help to remove the particulate matter from smoke, but tests show no improvement in ciliary defense response to filter cigarettes. It is also not known how long the effect lasts on the cilia; this factor apparently is variable. We have evidence that the lung airway's resistance is increased after the smoking of a single cigarette for approximately one hour. There is possibly some relationship between the return of normal resistance of the airway and the recovery of the cilia. Since smoking is a repetitive habit, it is easy to see that recovery can hardly take place before the drug is reapplied. Fortunately, our body defenses remain reasonably good, for once again we are supplied with a considerable reserve. Mucus excretion, cough, and the fact that there is a lack of uniform distribution of smoke throughout the lung means that certain cilia do recover, and the pulmonary toilet, although less efficient, does survive these initial insults. As the days change to weeks and the weeks extend to years, eventually the drugs carried by the smoke exert a telling effect on the cilia in more permanent ways. The cilia recover from the effect of the drug only when the smoker sleeps. By the time the smoker awakens, the cilia are active and mucus is present; the early morning cough of the chronic bronchitis patient is characteristic and again a helpful defense mechanism. However, as soon as the smoker has had his morning cough and has either spit out the mucus or swallowed it, he is aware of a deep tickling or irritating sensation in the throat as the cilia try to recover and attempt to remove more debris from the lung. The smoker interprets this as a need for a cigarette; thereupon the cilia are immediately put back to sleep, and our patient is now ready to accumulate further secretions and to breathe in and retain our atmospheric garbage for another day. Dr. Harold Levine of the Hines Veterans Hospital, who has furnished me almost as much material as the Federal government, defines the severe chronic bronchitic as the patient who must cough and spit before he can empty his bladder in the morning.

The relationship between industrial air pollution, emphysema, and cigarette smoking is now beginning to develop with a degree of rationality. It has been reported that smokers have four times the incidence of pulmonary emphysema in St. Louis as smokers in Winnepeg, Canada. This should be no surprise to anyone reading the previous paragraph. The smoker can certainly develop emphysema from particles drawn into his lungs from cigarettes alone. If we add to that the large amount of particulate matter that is dumped into the air from industrial waste, automobiles, and aircraft, the bronchial obstructive possibilities become multiplied. In addition, many of these particles brought in from the outside will carry tiny amounts of sulfurous or nitrous acid that, in themselves, may destroy lung tissue. These same particles, this same industrial air pollution brought into the tracheal bronchial tree of the nonsmoker, should be cleared away by his natural uninhibited defense mechanism. Of course air pollution is bad—it kills, but it kills primarily smokers.

The thing that is amazing to most of us is that the destructive effect of particulate inhalation does not destroy the lung even faster. The 1 to 2 per cent loss in lung function per year for smokers is an exceedingly important figure to remember. A boy who starts smoking at 15 has an excellent opportunity of being a respiratory cripple by the time he reaches his mid-forties. The one thing that may be important in permitting people to survive despite their habit is that most smokers intermittently try to stop. They may go a week or a month or perhaps even longer trying to break the habit. It is during those periods that there is some recovery on the part of the lung. There is also a great deal of difference in the way people smoke. One person may take one puff, then let the cigarette sit in the ashtray, while the next person inhales deeply every possible wisp of smoke that is available.

We do know that these processes become irreversible. After the cilia have lain dormant for long periods of time and the mucus load being cleared by means of coughing alone becomes relatively great, small tears or ulcerations occur in the bronchial mucosa, and the cells that contain the cilia are destroyed and expectorated with the rest of the mucus. New epithelium grows into the areas where it has been lost or shed earlier. This may not be quite the same as the original epithelial cells. The process is repeated over and over. Eventually a small continuing or chronic ulcer may develop, or some of the new type of epithelium that is encouraged to grow here may be of an abnormal type. At this point we have started cancer of the lung.

Cancer of the Lung

The relationship between cancer of the lung and chronic obstructive pulmonary disease is quite striking. We rarely see cancer of the lung in a patient who is entirely free of either bronchitis or emphysema. It is definitely possible to see chronic bronchitis and pulmonary emphysema in patients who do not have cancer. The fact that the two diseases go together is not surprising when we consider the positive factors we have discussed in the previous section. I have been involved actively in medicine for 25 years which, from a historical standpoint, is a relatively short period of time. However, I can say without doubt that two dramatic events have occurred in medicine in my quarter century of experience. One is the decreased incidence of poliomyelitis, and the other is the sad but unfortunately true increased incidence of cancer of the lung. As nearly as I can determine from statistical charts, in that period the mortality rate has tripled from this single disease process. American Cancer

Society data shows a 14 fold increase in male mortality in the past 40 years. Only pulmonary emphysema can challenge it from a percentage standpoint, and even here, in terms of total numbers, cancer of the lung is easily the winner among the killers in the respiratory tract. In 1967 our statistical data show that 54,407 persons died of cancer of the lung. Of this number, 9024 were females. This results in approximately a 5-to-1 preponderance of male to female deaths. As recently as 1955 cancer of the lung took the lives of 4100 women and 22,700 men. These specific data indicate the dramatic increase in incidence of this disease in both men and women. I recall very vividly during the days of my residency in radiology during the late 40's and early 50's that cancer of the lung was a relatively uncommon disease in our institution. We saw much more tuberculosis than carcinoma of the lung. The situation is now reversed. We have a diagnostic axiom in our department to the effect that, whenever there is a lesion in the lung and we do not have a specific diagnosis to offer, it is most likely cancer of the lung. This is true because cancer of the lung has become so common and because it manifests itself in many very devious ways.

It is amazing how many patients are brought into the hospital for convulsions or symptoms that point to the brain and, in the process of working up the patient for possible brain lesion, a chest film shows a large clearly identified mass that is a primary lung cancer. The whole ugly story rapidly unfolds. The patient's lung cancer was relatively asymptomatic except for the cough that the patient had already had for many years, and his only new symptom was an extension or metastasis to the brain. This patient is obviously not curable. Another type of presentation is the patient who has pulmonary emphysema and chronic shortness of breath and comes to the hospital because his shortness of breath has worsened. In the process of evaluating his chest, a mass appears that was not there on a previous study. We now know that the patient has undergone a malignant change in the lung; here again, we have a patient who cannot be operated on simply because he does not have enough lung function to survive. Many other types of patient presentations could be made that only emphasize the futility of this disease. If one counts every patient who has an established diagnosis of cancer of the lung, the five-year survival rate is approximately 7 per cent. If one alters the statistics to count only those who have primary lung tumors in the peripheral portion of the lung less than three-quarters of an inch in diameter and if at operation there is no evidence of spread beyond the initial site, the five-year survival rate is as high as 35 per cent. These may or may not be symptomatic.

On the basis of this, you may very logically ask if the outcome of the disease is not specifically related to the time of diagnosis. It would seem logical that, the earlier the diagnosis, the smaller the lesion and the more likely the chance of cure. This is certainly true of the peripherally placed primary malignancy. Most of these peripheral lesions are of a glandular type cell of origin to which we refer as adenocarcinoma, and this is the type of carcinoma that has been present in a relatively unchanging rate of occurrence for many generations. This is not the type of cancer of the lung that is showing the rapid increase in incidence and the rapid increase in American death rates. The malignant lesion that has given us so much trouble over the past 25 to 30 years is the neoplasm that arises in the bronchus. Its epithelial component is much like the epithelium of the skin and is referred to as oats cell (a descriptive term) or anaplastic (a term denoting rapid cell division) type cancer of the bronchus or lung. These are the tumors that are frequently associated with chronic bronchitis and pulmonary emphysema and are almost invariably associated with a history of smoking. The comparative incidence of this type of cancer of the lung in smokers and nonsmokers varies somewhat in the literature.

The Surgeon General's report of 1964, which was most critical of the use of tobacco, made an exhaustive survey of medical literature to that time and reported a 20 to 1 preponderance against tobacco and, in fact, offered some references of up to 70 to 1 when the types of tumor were taken into account. It is this, as well as the "mouse data" and other laboratory information, that led the Surgeon General to state that there is more than adequate evidence to assume that there is a causal relationship between smoking cigarettes and cancer of the lung. When such a strong statement is made by such a conservative source, it is difficult to understand why the actions of the public have not been more strongly influenced. As I have mentioned before, it is truly amazing that such inconsistencies as removing cyclamates from the market with relatively minimal data by suggesting they may produce malignancy can occur, and at the same time when there has been overwhelming evidence for over 10 years, that the cigarette industry is permitted to go relatively unchecked. The research into the effects of smoking on health continues at a tremendous rate. It requires a book larger than this simply to list the bibliographies of medical research work that is being done each year in this particular field. No one person can review all of this research work, but it can easily be sampled; if one takes the time and looks into the various studies that are being done, it becomes perfectly evident that this health habit is being condemned by 99 of 100 researchers. The tobacco industry maintains a research section. It constantly comes up with a few articles in favor of smoking, but these are so few in number and so overwhelmed by the rest of the medical data that they are, for the most part, lost except for what appears in tobacco literature. Since the industry cannot compete on a scientific basis with the medical community, it has appealed directly to the public with more and more glamor and social pressure in its advertising. This is the means by which it increased cigarette consumption to 572.6 billion cigarettes in 1967 and to 580 billion in 1973. Why worry about medical reports when you can get the public to identify your product with beauty, sex appeal, nature, masculinity, sports, and all forms of success?

I am sure that you are asking yourself, if all this medical literature is so overwhelming against cigarette smoking, why is it that some physicians still smoke? Most physicians who are still smoking acquired the habit when they were in high school and college and it is now a deeply ingrained habit. In addition to this, very few physicians spend any significant amount of time truly investigating the risk of this particular habit. Physicians, like other people, accept with a degree of casualness the statement that appears on every pack of cigarettes, "The Surgeon General Has Determined That Cigarette Smoking Is Dangerous to Your Health." As a group, they realize that there is an increased incidence of malignancy, emphysema, chronic bronchitis, and coronary heart disease with smoking, but very few have really investigated the degree to which this one habit can be implicated. The ones who have investigated the evidence and the ones who see patients with cancer of the lung in significant numbers, namely the radiologists and chest surgeons and chest medical specialists, have virtually abandoned smoking. One of the most interesting early studies on cancer of the lung and its relationship to smoking was carried out by British physicians on themselves. Their data resulted approximately as follows: if the physician lived in rural England and was a nonsmoker, he had no cancer of the lung. If he lived in London, where there was considerable air pollution, as a nonsmoker his chances of developing cancer of the lung were 1 in 256. If the physician smoked one pack of cigarettes per day and lived in London, his chances were 1 in 12 of developing cancer of the lung. If he lived in London and smoked 1½ packs per day, his chances of developing cancer of the lung were 1 in 6. British physicians were very much impressed with this data; within a very few years, 50 per cent of physicians who had been smoking prior to that time had stopped.

As a radiologist, I would like to make one more approach demonstrating to you the difficulty of the cancer of the lung problem. Let us assume that earlier diagnosis would result in more cures. Let us also assume that a chest X ray is one of our finer tools in making the diagnosis of cancer of the lung. Let us assume that it is possible to have, in a very convenient manner, a chest X ray every six months and that these films are examined by the most skillful radiologist. Therefore, if a chest X ray is negative at the first examination and shows some suspicion at the second examination, one would assume that this is a relatively early lesion and might have a better outlook than the general run of cancers of the lung seen by physicians in the hospital. Remember that we stated that those who come to the physician and hospital on a routine basis have a five-year survival rate of approximately 7 per cent. If a six-month chest X ray is offered and the patients are cooperative and examined carefully, those who develop the disease after the first film would be expected to have a significant increase in curability. A study in Philadelphia has been carried out in exactly this manner and has revealed that the cure rate changes from a lowly 7 per cent to a grand and glorious 9 per cent! We are, in effect, saying exactly what we might have anticipated from our earlier description of the pathogenesis of this disease. The lesion begins inside the bronchus and extends through the wall of the bronchus to lymph nodes and vascular structures before it ever develops a mass of sufficient size to be seen on the radiograph. If you wish to have a disease that puts you in the loser's category before the fight begins, cancer of the lung should be your choice.

It is interesting to note that the increasing incidence of cancer of the lung occurs in women as well as in men. The incidence of this disease seems to have increased with considerable rapidity in the last ten years. It may be that we are just entering the upswing of the incidence of cancer of the lung in females now as we faced it in males in 1945. This is no surprise to most of us, since it is an accepted fact that cigarette consumption by females has increased dramatically in the last 20 years. The development of cancer of the lung increases with the quantity of cigarettes consumed and with the susceptibility of the patient. As I implied in the study by British physicians, more than one pack of cigarettes a day carries a very high risk. Probably a better term for quantitating tobacco consumption is the term "pack years." One pack year is meant to imply that the patient smokes one pack of cigarettes a day for a year. Two-pack years could be one pack a day for two years or two packs a day for one year. Any patient who has reached the 30-pack-year category is in a high-risk group. If one stops to consider, 30-pack years can be reached at a relatively early age if one starts to smoke in one's teens. There seems to be little doubt that, as the female portion of our population increases its cigarette consumption, the female mortality rate from cancer of the lung will approach that of males. The statistical evidence now developing seems to confirm this impression. Those of us who are very concerned over the health of the public can watch the female increasing her cigarette consumption, and as we watch her increasing mortality rate we can truly say "You've come a long way, baby."

XIII. Decades of Degeneration or Distinction - Ages 65-74 and 75-84

The years of retirement, the years of leisure, "the last of life, for which the first was made," the lonely years, all are phrases that have been used to describe life after retirement. Note that I said life after retirement, not the time of growing old, for I do not know when people grow old. It varies tremendously with the person. Some people are old at 35, others die young in their late 80's. No one knows exactly why or how age affects different people in different ways. Most of us are quite certain that vital organs and their blood supply and physical activity play a very important role in maintaining vigor. There is no question that genetic background also is important. If all of the harmful influences that threaten our health could be eliminated, genetic influence would be the final criterion determining our span of life. However, everyone's genetic makeup is such that he would live many years beyond the average if that were the only limiting factor. The exceptions to the previous statement are obvious. We made them early in the text. There are genetically transferred diseases that greatly shorten life. However, persons with these genetic disorders do not reach the decades we are now approaching. Some persons insist that the life span of their ancestors is the most important contributor to their length of life. Securing data to prove or disprove this is difficult. However, most of us doubt if a good genetic background will protect us against all of the health hazards we have discussed. Good genes may only mean that one's parents may attend your funeral.

Our original goal was to find 100,000 deaths in the population under the age of 65 that could be deferred. We will count up the score in the summary.

Deferring death in the population over 65 is still a desirable goal and one that may be accomplished readily. Established physical fitness programs should be continued. If a person at this time of life has never participated in a physical fitness program, its adoption must be done with care. It should probably be limited to walking. However, physiologists have been surprised at how well people in their late years can condition themselves. It is not uncommon for men in their late years who are conditioned clearly to outperform men of half their age. Most notable of the examples is the highly publicized San Francisco waiter who recently died of cancer. He was 106 years of age, and had worked every day until the last 6 months of his life. He ran six miles per day and walked to work. He had been clocked at 17 seconds for the 100 yards. Not many American males in their 50's or even in their 30's can perform so vigorously. The best advice that can be given to the person who enters this golden decade is to keep active. This means both physical and mental activity. In this way one not only defers death, but adds zest and vitality to the years of living. Remember that more people rust out than wear out.

The three leading causes of death in present decades of interest have not changed from those in the 55-to-64 decade. You will notice that there is some shuffling of disorders that produce the fourth, fifth, and sixth highest death rates in these two decades. In the age group 75-to-84, accidents become the number-four killer, replacing emphysema and bronchitis, which were in the number four position in the age group 65 to 74. Of the overall leading causes of death, only cirrhosis of the liver and homicide show a decreasing death rate in the 75-to-84 age group compared to the decade earlier.

In 1967, 11,678,000 persons in our population were aged 65 to 74. Therefore, if you wish to obtain the approximate deaths for each of these entities, multiply the death rate listed in the chart by 117. In 1967, 5,945,000 persons in our population were between the ages of 75 and 84. If you wish to obtain the approximate number of deaths of each of the entities listed, multiply the death rate given by 60. We shall not make a chart of the leading causes of death for people over the age of 84; however, you may be interested to know that there were 1,174,000 people over the age of 84 in 1967.

Cancer

In 1967 malignancy took the lives of 310,983 Americans. Of that number of deaths, 155,304, almost exactly one half, occurred in persons in the age group between 65 and 84. Cancer takes lives in every age group, but it takes its largest toll in the late decades of life.

It is not uncommon for people to consider cancer as a single disease. I wish to correct that concept immediately. The term cancer or malignant disease implies only that there are cells that are multiplying out of control and that these cells are abnormal to the body. This is true for all types of malignancy; however, we stated earlier that we normally describe malignancies in reference to the organ from which these abnormal cells originated. Therefore, a cancer of the kidney and a cancer of the lung would affect two entirely different types of cells. Since the cells of origin are different, these malignancies act differently and have an entirely different outlook. The next complicating step is that every organ has several different types of cells. Therefore, a cancer of the kidney may be of several different types. To complicate the picture further, the abnormal or malignant cell will differ from the cell of origin in varying degrees. The more the cancer cell resembles the cell of origin, the less apt it is to be a rapidly growing or a wild type of tumor. You can now see that, if we are speaking of a cancer of the lung, we must ask what is the cell of origin and in addition what is the degree of maturation of the malignant cell compared to the cell of origin. All of these features enter into the behavioral characteristics of the tumor and as such enter into the treatment plans and the results that can be expected.

Tremendous amounts of information regarding cancer have been reported by clinicians and researchers in the last decade. Most medical libraries can supply endless references on all phases of malignant disease. Most of this is very complicated. I would suggest, if you have specific questions in regard to malignant disease, that you contact your physician or the American Cancer Society in your city or state. Government information is not as readily available as that which can be supplied by the American Cancer Society. In addition, local cancer societies usually have responsible physicions to whom they can turn for specific advice or recommendation.

There are some fundamental features about cancer that I feel are important to mention here. In addition, there are some other facts that I think you will find interesting, and these can certainly stimulate thoughts about this very complex disease. People are inclined to express impatience with physicians for not having found a cause for cancer. Since cancer is many different diseases, it is very likely that there are many different causes. We have already mentioned the fact that the Surgeon General has implicated cigarettes as a cause of lung cancer, yet we know that not everyone who has a long and heavy smoking history develops cancer of the lung. We also know that a few nonsmokers develop cancer of the lung. Usually the cancer of the lung in the nonsmoker is of a somewhat different variety. Thus, there is an underlying implication that a second factor must be present. This factor is usually indicated as a "host" factor. What we are really saying is that there are different degrees of susceptibility to cancer in different people. This may have a genetic basis. We know that some families are remarkably free of cancer; we also know of other families in which this disease takes an unusual toll. Therefore, some type of familial or genetic factor must exist. If the previous predisposing factor is present and established, then a precipitating factor, which in the case of carcinoma of the lung or larynx may be cigarette smoke, combines with this predisposing factor to produce the malignant lesion. We also know that the host factor plays a very important role even after the malignancy develops. There are some persons who seem to tolerate malignant disease very well and in whom the maligant lesion grows very slowly, probably because of resistance on the part of the host. At the same time, other victims of the disease seem to offer no resistance to the tumor and what clinically and microscopically may look like a relatively slow growing malignancy. In such a patient the disease may be fatal in a very short period of time. We have, therefore, added one more intangible to the many other facets of this disease, all of which make prediction of the outcome difficult.

A great deal of work has been done on the relationship of viral infections to cancer. It is not uncommon to see in magazines or newspapers reports that viruses cause malignancy. Unless you read the article carefully and go into it further, you may be seriously misled. Most of us think of viruses as causing infections such as colds and measles or mumps, all of which are contagious, and our first thought is that cancer must be a contagious disease—a frightening thought. Our hope is that, since some viral diseases, mainly polio, are now being prevented by immunization, there must be forthcoming an immunization against cancer. One can conjure both hope and fear from the same source. First, on the matter of contagion, to my knowledge there has never been an example of a patient spreading malignancy to another person. I can conceive of some exceptions to that statement. For instance, if a person were to receive a kidney with a small focus of cancer as a transplanted organ and if the kidney transplant were successful, it is also possible that cancer could grow. In this sense, one person could donate a malignant disease to another. To my knowledge no such case has ever occurred. I am offering this only as a theoretical concept of how tumor cells might be spread; at the same time, I am making the point that, in the usual context of human experience, cancer is not a contagious disease.

Viruses, as etiological agents for cancer, are extremely attractive. Viruses have certainly been related to laboratory malignancies in animals and have also been implicated in forms of cancer in chickens. Vaccines against these laboratory cancers have been reported to be reasonably effective. A relationship of viruses to human cancer has not been established, although many scientists are very enthusiastic about the possible relationship between viruses and human malignancy. One theory is that the virus enters the cell and becomes involved in the chemistry of the gene; it may alter the ribonucleic (RNA) or deoxyribonucleic (DNA) acid of the gene itself. It is felt that this genetic alteration may play an important part in the host factor that we have described above. Others feel that the viral cancer relationship in humans is a more direct one, and there is some interesting and somewhat startling evidence to offer in regard to this relationship. For instance, cancer of the penis occurs four to six times as frequently in uncircumcised as in circumcised males. Cancer of the penis is also more common in males who have or have had syphilis. The implication is that a subtle, possibly low-grade infection, most likely viral, exists in the environment provided by the lack of circumcision or previous disease. Similar statistics indicate that virgin females do not develop cancer of the cervix. At the same time cancer of the cervix appears to be more common in the female who is sexually active, especially if sexual activity began early in life. Cancer of the cervix rarely occurs in females whose husbands are circumcised. Again, the implication would be that some type of low-grade infection, possibly viral in origin, is presented to the cervix by the male and that cancer of the cervix results. In this sense, cancer of the cervix may be considered a venereal disease. I would hasten to add that no one has ever demonstrated a virus as definite etiology in human malignancy. Epidemiological evidence of a viral etiology of cancer is suggested when a large number of cases appear in a given locality. The acute leukemia found among children in Niles, Illinois from 1957 to 1960 is a case in point. However, even such clusters must be examined carefully, for even with a random incidence of disease, some clustering is bound to occur. In addition to this, when clusters occur in families, one must assume that there is a genetic role. There is still another theory relating viruses to cancer. This states that the virus involved in cancer is a common one, and that it occurs in all of us. It produces cancer only when host factors change. In this sense, we may in the future identify a number of risk factors, just as we now do in coronary heart disease. These factors would be those that change host resistance or increase the virility of the virus.

The supposed role of the virus in malignant disease is indeed an exciting one. Time alone will tell us whether its relationship can be used in any way to prevent the disease. At best, proof of the relationship and the development of a vaccine are many years away.

Other epidemiological considerations offer some insight into malignant behavior. For instance, in this country there has been a steady decrease in the incidence of cancer of the stomach. The same holds true for most European countries. Despite this, cancer of the stomach has been increasing in Japan and Iceland. At the same time, cancer of the colon is showing a relatively slow increase among Americans and Europeans, while the incidence is extremely low in Orientals. These facts tend to emphasize the possible relationship between dietary habits and the development of malignant disease. It is known that when Japanese immigrate to Hawaii or California, the incidence of cancer of the colon increases until it matches the incidence of Americans. It is also true that their incidence of cancer of the stomach tends to decrease when they live in this country; this may occur in the first generation. It is also known that cancer of the nasal pharynx is much more common in Chinese than Americans and that, even with immigration of the Chinese to America, the incidence of this type of cancer remains 20 to 30 times as great in that group as in the American population. This would imply, in contrast to intestinal-tract malignancies, that there is a racial or genetic tendency that is unchanged by environment among the Chinese.

There are, in addition to these differences in nationalities and races, certain correlations and lack of correlations that occur between different disease processes. It has been reported that diabetics have fewer malignancies than nondiabetics. There is, however, one glaring exception to this rule. This is carcinoma of the body of the uterus, which occurs in females who are obese and usually diabetics. There is a moderate increase in cancer of the biliary tract in patients who are obese. Pernicious anemia, which results in atrophy of the gastric mucosa, leads toward an increased incidence of cancer of the stomach. Scleroderma (a disease of the skin and its supporting tissues) is associated with an increased incidence of cancer of the esophagus. Ulcerative colitis (probably because of chronic irritation) creates a high incidence of cancer of the colon. Cancer of the gallbladder rarely occurs in patients who do not have gallstones. Here again the malignancy probably develops as a response to chronic irritation. Polyps of the colon, particularly those that are of the familial type, cause a high incidence of malignancies of that organ.

As we identify more precipitating and predisposing factors of malignancy, prevention of this disease can become more sensible. Medical advice can be based upon the predicted rate of malignant occurrence. We know, for instance, that familial polyps of the colon have a nearly 100 per cent incidence of malignancy if they are not removed. Therefore colectomy is advised as soon as the diagnosis is made. In other diseases where the incidence of the malignant complication is not so great, the patient can be seen and reevaluated at frequent intervals. If a precipitating factor can be identified, the patient certainly must be advised to avoid that agent. This is one more reason why all patients are advised to avoid cigarette smoking. The risks of asbestos in the air are now realized; there is apparently a high correlation betwen the inhalation of asbestos particles and the development of tumors of the pleura. It has been known for years that certain dye compounds result in cancer of the bladder. These specific precipitating factors in malignancy can be identified and should be avoided. We can only hope that more of them can be identified in the future and that patients will listen to our advice more attentively than they have done with regard to avoiding cigarette smoke.

Cancer Control

There is a distinct difference between cancer prevention and cancer control. Cancer prevention is, of course, ideal, but until we can identify all precipitating factors or can immunize against the predisposing or host factors, we must be content to work on projects of cancer control. Control implies that the patient already has the disease and that it is being adequately treated. The American Cancer Society estimates that at least one fourth and probably as high as one third of all cancer deaths could be avoided if the diagnosis were made while the disease was localized to the involved organ. There is certainly a high degree of truth in these estimates. The types of malignancy most difficult to diagnose are those with the poorest outlook. We have already discussed the problems of cancer of the lung and have indicated that in most instances it has spread to the regional nodes or bloodstream by the time the patient presents to his physician. We have also indicated the limitations of the chest X ray in making an early diagnosis of cancer of the lung. Other diagnostic techniques offer some potential; microscopic examination of the sputum may on occasion be helpful, but is quite time-consuming. However, as we have indicated on repeated occasions, cancer of the lung is a preventable disease. Some 90 to 95 per cent of cancer of the lung occurs in those people who have, by their own choice, ignored all of the scientific evidence available and have continued to smoke cigarettes.

Energy can be more fruitfully exerted in the areas where physical examination can identify early lesions. Cancers of the skin and cancers of the oral and rectal cavities are areas where early diagnoses are accompanied by a high rate of cure. Therefore, it is only a matter of bringing the patient and the physician together.

Mass laboratory surveys for cancer detection hold great popular appeal. Good results have come from the use of Pap smears to identify early lesions of the cervix. Cancer of the cervix apparently exists for a relatively long period of time as a premalignant lesion. It is at this point that it can be identified from the smears; when treated in the premalignant stage, the cure rate approaches 100 per cent. One can find varying degrees of optimism in the literature with regard to these Pap smear surveys. A Canadian group reported in 1968 that there has been no improvement from mortality of carcinoma of the cervix that could be related to the screening techniques. Other reports are much more optimistic; certainly, the impressions gained by gynecologists and radiologists are to the effect that there has been an important change in the occurrence of advanced cancer of the cervix. Most of us feel very strongly about the value of screening smears—it has been one of the most important measures in cancer control in the past fifteen years. It is important that one word of caution be offered at this point. The Pap smear on a "do-it-yourself" basis has been reported to give as high as 50 per cent false negatives. It is likely that if all females were to collect their own Pap smears, the yield would be far too low to be acceptable. Pap tests must be done by a physician or his assistant so that the specimen can be collected properly.

The examination of the female breast is another area where early diagnosis offers considerable reward. There is apparently no obvious premalignant lesion to compare with that seen in the cervix. In contrast to cancer of the cervix, breast malignancy is more common in the female virgin or at least in the female who has never been pregnant. Breast tissue is characteristically irregular, which makes detection of small malignancies difficult. X ray examination of the breast adds to the accuracy of the breast examination; however, it is time-consuming and results in considerable radiation exposure of the breast. We know of no ill effect from local irradiation to the breast, but as part of good radiological practice, we recommend that it be done only on patients when there is a high risk or in patients with questionable physical findings, with or without symptoms of malignancy. Females should examine their own breasts; if there is a change or an area that seems unusual, the physician should be consulted.

The radiologist plays multiple roles in the general spectrum of cancer. The radiologist is the clinicians' first consultant in the diagnosis of those malignancies that lie beyond the vision of the eye or the touch of the finger. This includes all the malignancies of the gastrointestinal tract except those of the rectum and low colon and those of the mouth. It is true that the stomach can be examined with the gastroscope, but the gastroscope is rarely used as a primary diagnostic instrument; it is used principally when there are X ray changes that require additional confirmation. The X ray is the primary diagnostic tool in cancer of the lung, brain, kidney, and bone. It is also used to help evaluate the extent and spread of virtually all other malignancies. Without the use of the X ray, diagnostic medicine would be much the same as it was at the turn of the century. In addition to the radiological role in diagnosis of cancer, X ray therapy is the method of choice for certain types of malignancy. This is particularly true of cancer of the cervix in the female, cancer of the lymphatic tissues, particularly Hodgkins' disease, and some of the tumors of nerve origin in children. It is used in conjunction with surgery in other conditions and as a palliative measure when surgery has failed in other forms of neoplastic disease.

Even with the radiologist's extensive role in cancer diagnosis and treatment, he is frequently asked if X ray diagnostic procedure might not induce or spread malignancy in the patient. These questions are asked by patients who have seen newspaper or magazine articles equating the incidence of leukemia with radiation exposure. There is little doubt that radiation can induce malignancy under the proper circumstances. For instance, we know that the incidence of cancer of the thyroid is increasing in children who have been irradiated for problems of the thymus gland. This is why radiation to the thymus is no longer considered a generally acceptable procedure. Apparently the thyroid in the infant is very susceptible to radiation changes. The radiation dose to the thyroid in these instances was relatively low, but was still in the area of 300 to 900 units. I recall having seen a patient in his early 30's who had a malignant bone tumor arising from the maxillary sinus. This patient's history was that some 15 years earlier he had had a malignant tumor in the nasopharynx and had been heavily radiated. The nasopharyngeal tumor had been cured, but the second malignancy had formed in the area of the radiation beam. The patient was fortunate to survive his first tumor and live long enough to develop the second. Physicians associated with the case felt that the second tumor had been very probably induced by radiation.

The first evidence that radiation might produce malignant tumors was reported in the early 1900's. This followed the development of skin cancer in the hands of radiation workers. This was one of the hazards of being a radiologist in the early years of this specialty. We have since learned that not only X rays induce skin malignancy; radiation from the sun can also do so. I am sure you have read, and it seems to be a well established fact, that chronic exposure to the sun's rays can produce malignant degeneration of the skin.

The effects of total body irradiation such as occurred at Hiroshima and Nagasaki have been studied extensively; the results of these studies are quite complicated. However, there appears to be an increased incidence of leukemia in those patients who were exposed. The incidence of leukemia seems to be higher in patients who had large doses than in those who had small exposure. The International Commission on Radiological Protection tried to take the Japanese data and extrapolate the dosage downward to a point where it would be comparable to the dose received in diagnostic X ray studies. They have calculated that, for every million people who undergo diagnostic X ray examination, one or two additional cases of leukemia develop each year for approximately 13 years. Since the incidence of leukemia is between 50 and 60 patients per million per year, it is difficult to know whether we will even be able accurately to identify the one or two additional cases that may theoretically occur. It is not my intent to defend diagnostic radiology as a harmless tool, although I feel that it is criticized for sensational reasons from time to time. The above data seem to put radiation in a more proper perspective. One must always weigh the values to be gained against the potential risk. In this instance, although the risks are present, they are small, and the benefits to be gained from early diagnosis of malignancy or even the demonstration of the fracture or infection seems far to outweigh the risk involved.

We are particularly careful to avoid total body exposure. This is especially true of children. Certainly, the basic reason for our profession is to eliminate disease, not create it. Professionals in the field practice good radiological safety procedures.

Malignancies of the colon and rectum have a high curability rate when diagnosed early. Early lesions in these areas should be between 60 and 80 per cent curable. In 1967 there were 43,513 deaths from malignancy of the colon and rectum. Not all of these could have been prevented, some patients did not develop the symptoms until the disease was widespread, and it is not practicable to do a barium enema X ray on every person over the age of 45. However, the rectum can be examined easily with the finger, and most of the lesions in the rectum and lower colon can be felt or seen with direct vision using the proctosigmiodoscope. Bleeding from the rectum or changes in bowel habits are more than adequate reason to see your physician; unless he has some obvious explanation, an X ray examination of the colon should be obtained.

Cancer as a whole is the responsibility of the individual and the physician. Some of my physician colleagues have been deemphasizing the value of the routine annual physical. From the standpoint of cancer detection, this is unfortunate. It is granted that many patients are seen and that the yield of disease is relatively low. However, the success rates with early malignancies, particularly in the previously designated areas are good enough to warrant it. There seems to be little doubt that portions of the routine annual physical might be carried out by assistants, but the responsibility for examination of the areas indicated will still be up to the examining physician. With the help of assistants and history forms filled out by the patient, the Sloan Kettering Program makes it possible for one physician carefully to evaluate 60 patients a day. His degree of suspicion and evaluation of the overall risk factors will determine the extent of the more specialized examination needed. The chest X ray, laboratory examination of the urine, and the barium enema are the most usual next steps in the search for a diagnosis.

If no arrangements for an annual physical can be made, the next cancer control measure is seeing a physician when symptoms appear. A very satisfactory percentage of malignancies can be cured at the onset of symptoms. There are some notable exceptions, but these should not deter you from seeking medical advice in the presence of symptoms. Of those patients who see their physician late, the reasons for the delay are usually based on emotional fears or misconceptions or misinterpretations of their symptoms. These misconceptions and emotional restraints cut across all social and educational levels; one of the most common reasons given for delay in appearance for medical care relates to fear. Patients are afraid of physicians and hospitals. It is not an uncommon story for a patient to tell her physician that she was aware of the mass or the complaint for some time, but that she was afraid that the lesion might be malignant. She therefore felt that, as long as she did not know for sure, she would be happier not knowing that she had a disease. Such an attitude implies that all cancers are incurable. This is far from the truth. Cure rates depend on the organ involved, the extent of the disease when the patient is first seen, and the growth rate of the tumor. Neither you nor I have any control over the organ involved. You as a patient have moderate control over the stage of the disease at the time you appear. Unfortunately, you do not have total control, since there are some deep-seated, unknown, asymptomatic lesions. We as physicians have the responsibility to make the diagnosis as early as possible. This depends upon your presentation, upon the organ involved, and the accessibility of that organ to our diagnostic tools. Some of us have rested some hope in the development of a cancer-seeking radioactive isotope. This offers a theoretically ideal diagnostic tool. With such a tool we could inject a radioactive material, wait for it to find the malignant tissue, identify it, and see that the proper treatment was instituted. Unfortunately, such radioactive materials are not available, although some are showing limited degrees of promise.

It is not my intent to discuss the future of medicine in malignant disease. Our role here is to find preventable deaths. The American Cancer Society tells me that there should have been nearly 100,000 preventable cancer deaths in 1967. I think this is worth considering. The most important advice I can offer you is to develop an optimistic attitude about malignancy. Do not avoid your physician because of fears. Learn all you can about the disease from the many sources available. Seek medical help on a routine basis if possible, and seek it without delay if symptoms do develop.

Strokes

One of the components of major cardiovascular renal disease is vascular disease of the central nervous system. All vascular lesions of the central nervous system are clumped together under the single term "strokes." Vascular diseases of the central nervous system represent the third largest cause of death in the United States. As a killer, they trail only heart disease and cancer. In 1967, 202,184 deaths were attributed to strokes. It is of interest to note that, of this large number, only 36,761 occurred in patients under the age of 65 years. When we review the decades from 65 through 84, we find that strokes took 123,194 lives during this 20-year interval. It is apparent that stroke is primarily a disease of the elderly.

It is true that vascular disease of the central nervous system is influenced by the same risk factors that we have discussed with heart disease. These risk factors are once again: elevated blood cholesterol, elevated blood pressure, cigarette smoking, obesity, and sedentary living. The most important of these is high blood pressure. Hypertensive patients with electrocardiographic changes have a nine times greater risk of stroke than normatensive patients with normal electrocardiographic studies. There is one very striking difference between the brain as a target organ compared to the heart. The oxygen consumption of the brain remains surprisingly constant at all times; certainly, the blood flow to the brain is maintained at virtually a constant level. There are, of course, exceptions to the previous statement, depending upon the presence of disease. However, the brain apparently demands very little more oxygen when it is being used in a very strenuous manner than it does during rest or even sleep. It cannot demand and does not need additional oxygen as the heart must have additional oxygen during periods of stress. The factors that limit the blood flow to the brain are primarily those of the vessels and their resistance. Flow changes may be caused by a plaque in a major artery at its point of bifurcation or, as is the case with high blood pressure, there may be changes in the caliber and distensibility of the peripheral vessels. It seems that increased blood pressure drives the vascular disease changes farther down into smaller and smaller vessels. Because of the inherent differences between the brain and the heart, vascular disease kills by damaging the brain at a period some 10 to 20 years later in life than coronary vascular disease.

We certainly do not imply that there are no mechanisms by which the blood flow to the brain can be altered. The blood supply to the brain is critical. The brain, while it represents only 2 per cent of the body's total weight, receives one sixth of the total cardiac output of blood and uses nearly 20 per cent of the oxygen supply of the entire body. It is easy to imagine that the designer of such a system would arrange for certain checks, balances, and safety devices by which this high blood flow and high oxygen supply could be maintained. For instance, we know that if a person inhales 5 per cent carbon dioxide, this will serve as a very potent dilator of the cerebral vessels, and the blood flow may be increased as much as 75 per cent. Other drugs are less effective in producing increased cerebral blood flow. Therefore, it would seem that nature has provided the brain with a great protective mechanism against the accumulation of carbon dioxide. We also know that, when a patient is anemic, the blood flow to the brain in cubic centimeters per minute is increased; conversely, if the patient has too many red cells, the blood flow through the brain appears to be slowed. All of these mechanisms are directed toward maintaining an adequate oxygen supply to the central nervous system. Fainting is a protective mechanism. If blood flow to the brain is reduced, a person will faint; when a person faints, he falls or assumes a horizontal position, which increases cerebral blood flow, and the person recovers from the faint.

The blood supply to the brain is through four major vessels: the two carotid arteries, one on either side of the neck, and the two vertebral arteries, which extend posteriorly along the vertebral bodies. These vessels tend to unite with each other as they enter the base of the brain; therefore, if blood flow in any one of these vessels is decreased, the others tend to compensate for this loss. Here again nature has tried to create a protective type of circulation to the brain. The system would seem to be better than the one we have in the heart, and these features also aid in delaying the age of onset of cerebral vascular disease. However, a significant number of people have anatomic anomalies of these vessels, and it is thought that these may predispose to arteriosclerosis and strokes. These anomalies have their origin during embryonic life and cannot be altered by persons or physicians. A study correlating these anatomical changes and strokes would be of interest and possibly be valuable in predicting brain vascular disease.

It is also true that some sections of the brain are more vulnerable to oxygen shortage than others. It has been reported that the cortex of the brain, or the superficial portion of it, may be irreparably damaged after five minutes of anoxia. However, the medulla, or brain stem, may recover after as much as 30 minutes of anoxia. I am sure it will come as no surprise to you when I indicate that the medulla carries out the basic functions of breathing, involuntary intestinal motility, and even to a moderate degree control of the heart rate and rhythm. These are the most basic functions of life. They are, therefore, the most protected. The cortex of the brain, which is involved with memory, judgment, intelligence, motor functions, and sensory reactions in the body, is less vital to life and more complex in its engineering and is, therefore, the least protected or more vulnerable to oxygen loss. We have now offered some logical reason why elderly persons are forgetful and show personality changes; even speech or motor alterations occur long before brain deterioration threatens life. Over and over again we have made the statement that any organ functions well so long as it is receiving an adequate blood supply. This is certainly true of the heart, lungs, liver, kidneys, and it should be even more apparent in our discussion of the brain.

Approximately two thirds of the catastrophic events that we commonly refer to as strokes are caused by obstruction of a significant cerebral vessel. There are several mechanisms by which the cerebral vessel can become occluded. Multiple arteriosclerotic plaques in the carotid and vertebral vessels may reduce the total blood flow to the brain to a point where circulation is sluggish and intravascular clotting occurs. This may occur as part of the aging process. It may happen more acutely if the patient has been existing on marginal cerebral blood flow for some time and his life then becomes complicated by a drop in blood pressure. Such a drop in blood pressure can occur if the patient has a myocardial infarction or if the patient loses blood through trauma or other internal blood loss. In such an event the stiff vessels can no longer dilate to compensate for the reduced number of circulating red cells. The brain suffers reduced blood supply, and rapid deterioration of the central nervous system results. Blood pressure drops also may occur with anesthetic agents. Anesthesiologists are all aware of the possibility that strokes will complicate a necessary operation in an elderly patient. Regardless of precautions, strokes too often still complicate operative procedures.

Clots may form in small intracerebral vessels simply on the basis of sluggish flow through these vessels. Another mechanism by which clots can occlude a cerebral vessel is the so-called "embolic phenomenon." This implies that the clot was formed elsewhere, as in the carotid vessel; it is broken off and is carried upstream, where it lodges in another smaller vessel to produce cerebral infarction. By far the most common mechanism creating emboli in the brain involves the deposition of platelets and clot formation on the atheromatous plaques in the carotid vessels. Carotid vessels frequently are the site of such plaques; since these produce eddy currents that alter the flow characteristics, the tiny platelet particles in the blood tend to stick to the plaque and thus form a clot that later serves as an embolus to the cerebral vessels. One fine preventive measure exists here—aspirin prevents platelet stickiness, thereby reducing clots. Laboratory data are good. Clinical trials are underway. Unless there is some reason why you cannot take aspirin (tendency to intestinal bleeding or allergy) two aspirins a week may serve as a real stroke preventive. It may also be helpful in the heart.

It is also known that the heart itself may serve as a site in forming clots, which are later carried to the brain. This is especially true of persons who have tumors that arise in the heart. These are rare; cerebral emboli may be the first symptoms of such a tumor. It is also true that if the heart has dysrhythmic contractions (auricular fibrillation) particularly when caused by valvular disease, clots may form in some of the segments that are not contracting normally. These clots may later embolize the brain.

There are some opportunities for preventive measures regarding the thromboembolic type of strokes other than aspirin. For instance, if we can prove that a source of emboli may be an ulcerated plaque in a vessel outside of the cranial vault, this may represent a surgically correctable lesion. Vascular surgery has become a mature art, and a localized lesion of this type lends itself very well to surgical correction. It is apparent that, if the stroke has already occurred, repair of the vessel will be of limited value. It is, therefore, a major medical diagnostic problem for physicians to identify patients who may have surgically remedial vascular lesions before brain injury occurs. Identification of these patients is difficult. The physician tries to identify them from the patient's history of repeated but completely recoverable cerebral vascular ischemic periods. He also tries to palpate the difference of the pulses on each side of the neck. When the question of asymmetry of carotid pulses arises, X ray studies of the vessels will be required for a more specific diagnosis.

Thromboembolic phenomena are the most common type of strokes. The other major category of catastrophic stroke is the intercranial hemorrhage. The brain is tightly enclosed in the skull, and adding free hemorrhage or a blood clot into this space very obviously compromises the brain. Intracranial hemorrhage implies that there has been a break or tear in a major artery. When this break in the blood vessel occurs inside the skull, but outside of the actual brain tissue itself, it is referred to as a subarachnoid hemorrhage. This type of hemorrhage accounts for approximately 12 per cent of all cerebral vascular accidents. As you may imagine, subarachnoid hemorrhages may result from a congenital weakness in a blood vessel. For this reason, this type of stroke tends to occur in a younger age group. Subarachnoid hemorrhages also occur from an acute elevation of blood pressure such as may occur with a toxemia of pregnancy. Here again a younger age group would be involved. Trauma may result in tearing of the vessels as they pass through the skull or tearing of small vessels as they penetrate the skull itself. This is another mechanism for producing subarachnoid hemorrhages.

Hemorrhage may also occur from blood vessels after they have penetrated the brain itself. This results in an intracerebral hemorrhage, or hematoma. This collection of blood will result in tearing and displacement of the brain locally.

This type of stroke accounts for approximately 20 per cent of cerebral vascular accidents. It is, therefore, somewhat more common than subarachnoid hemorrhage. This type of intracranial hemorrhage is primarily related to hypertension, less commonly to congenital malformations of the blood vessels within the brain itself. There are times when surgical evacuation of a clot can be lifesaving to the patient. Certainly, this is always a consideration, for otherwise the outcome of the patient's illness is predictably bad.

Whenever a patient with a cerebral vascular accident presents himself to the physician, an effort is made to classify the type of stroke that is present, whether it be hemorrhage or a thromboembolic phenomenon. In addition, a serious attempt is made to determine the localization of the stroke. It is well known to physicians, and perhaps to most of you, that certain areas of the brain carry out specific functions. You may not be aware of the fact that the right side of the brain controls the left side of the body. It is also true that if you are right-handed, the left side of your brain is the dominant hemisphere; because of this dominance, the left side will also contain the speech center. Using many anatomical and physiological bits of information, the neurologist or neurosurgeon can localize the area involved from the clinical evaluation of the patient. If there is any possibility of surgical intervention, brain scans, or X ray vascular studies, will be carried out. However, when the patient presents with sudden loss of use of the right arm and at the same time has lost the ability to speak, we know that there has been a stroke involving the motor strip and the speech center on the left.

If we are to find more preventive measures in the field of cerebral vascular diseases, we need to know more about the epidemiology of the disease. Dr. J. F. Kurtzke has devoted an entire book to the subject, *Epidemiology of Cerebral Vascular Disease*. He is convinced that there is only slight variation in the incidence of cerebral vascular disease in people of different races and nationalities. It is his impression that the only entity that correlates with cerebral vascular disease is aging. Many other authors feel that there is an unusually high incidence of stroke in the black race. This is apparently because of the high incidence of hypertension. As stated earlier, the presence of hypertension associated with electrocardiographic changes implying muscular stress of the heart increases the incidence of cerebral vascular accident by nine times. The influence of diabetes on arteriosclerosis also increases the incidence of cerebral vascular disease in this group of persons. However, all authors seem to agree that if we discuss strokes in patients under 60, the same risk factors that were discussed with heart disease are important here. This is especially true of hypertension. The prevention of significant hypertension is therefore an important point in reducing the number of strokes. It seems logical that a program that tends to slow the biological aging process would also be helpful in preventing strokes. Our program to prevent myocardial infarction is the best we have to offer. It is our hope that we can keep the vascular tree in such good condition that the peak age incidence of strokes can be moved from the 70's and 80's to the 80's and 90's. The importance of preventing cerebral vascular accidents becomes even more evident when survival statistics are surveyed. There is considerable variation in survival statistics, depending upon the age of the population surveyed and the extent of the cerebral vascular accident. Most series indicate that a patient having a significant stroke has less than a 10 per cent chance of surviving three years.

XIV. Summary

The first factual data that we presented to you involved the chart of the 15 leading causes of death in the United States for 1967. At this point, go back and look at the chart on page 303. All of these diseases should be more familiar now than when you first saw the chart. As you look at the chart for the second time, you will be reminded that the leading killer is heart disease. You will also notice that five of the leading 15 causes of death involve either the heart or the blood vessels. Since both of these are so closely related in both health and disease, we discussed them together.

Entry number 5 in the leading cause of death is listed as "Influenza and pneumonia except pneumonia in the newborn." We have said nothing about influenza, but have included it with pneumonia. In 1967, deaths from influenza were very small; they make up about 2 per cent of the deaths in this particular entry. There have been years when influenza epidemics were a major cause of death, but this has not been true for some time. In our discussions, pneumonia and influenza could be classed as models of infectious disease. Methods for preventing and treating pneumonia are the same as those for infectious disease in general.

Diabetes was the eighth leading cause of death in 1967. There have been some scattered remarks about this disease, but we offered no concentrated section about it for obvious reasons. There is no way of preventing diabetes.

Diabetes can be prevented only if all of the diabetic genotypes stop having children. Since about 70 per cent of our people are diabetic genotypes, this advice is impracticable. Since adult forms of diabetes are controllable, harsh preventive measures are worse than the disease. We know that, if a person who is potentially a diabetic becomes obese, his blood sugar will rise and sugar will be spilled in the urine. However, with weight reduction the metabolic processes return to normal. Therefore, this form of diabetes can be controlled relatively easily with diet. We also know that some diabetics develop their disease late in life and that it may be a product of the aging process.

A person who develops severe diabetes early in life (juvenile diabetes) is a different matter. These persons have a shortened life expectancy and suffer many of the complications of diabetes including loss of sight, vascular disease and renal failure. It has been estimated that there will be one million blind diabetics in the U. S. by 1980. Nature has a way of controlling the number of these patients in society by making it very difficult for them to conceive or to complete a pregnancy. However, the physician has entered the picture, and through improved control of their disease a certain number of these persons do become pregnant. The management of such pregnancy is a most difficult assignment. Most such cases are now handled by teams of physicians, including obstetricians, internists, and neonatologists. Even with the best of care the perinatal mortality rate runs about ten times as high in this group as in the nondiabetic group. Despite the high perinatal mortality, some of these children survive. Some have birth defects. Recently, we saw three children born with absence of the lumbar spine and lower spinal cord. This is an anomaly limited almost entirely to diabetics requiring and taking insulin. Other babies born of such mothers have problems with fluid balance and respiration. If one parent has diabetes, the infant has a 22 times greater chance of having diabetes than if both parents were nondiabetics. If both of his parents are diabetics, the child has a 60 times greater chance of having diabetes than if his parents were nondiabetics.

Since we strongly advocate quality children, we feel that all persons who are diabetic during the childbearing years should seek genetic counseling for individual advice. Both family histories and the severity of the diabetes should be considered. The number of juvenile diabetes cases can be reduced and the quality of infants improved if certain young diabetics refrain from having children. This would not eliminate all diabetes, but would eliminate some of the more disabling forms of the disease.

The tenth leading cause of death, "Other bronchial pulmonary diseases," you will recognize as pulmonary emphysema and chronic bronchitis. There are some other minor entries under this head, but emphysema has increased so rapidly that it dominates this entry. I hope that you have taken the opportunity to look at the ten-year trends and the death statistics of certain diseases of interest. This chart is number XXVIII on page 329.

As you review the leading causes of death and as you recall our discussions over the previous pages, you will be reminded that there are measures that can be used to reduce the death rate or prevent the disease in every category listed. It is therefore time for us to lay down the rules of survival by which we must live if we are to improve our lives, both quantitatively and qualitatively. We have already told you that, at age 60, a man has no greater life expectancy in this country than he had during the days of the Roman Empire. Women do considerably better. However, the evidence of the last few years implies that the life expectancy of the female is starting to decrease rather than increase. Physicians will continue research into methods of disease control and prevention, but it is clear that we, as physicians, are losing ground to the self-inflicted, the socially inflicted, and even the technigenic diseases of our era. Your survival and that of your family depends to a very large degree on how you plan your counterattack on the forces that threaten to increase our mortality rate.

Let me first list these rules.

1. Develop an attitude of self-preservation and relaxed confidence.

2. Develop a working relationship with your physician in regard to:
   (a) Physical checkups and specific health advice regarding cancer control and the early recognition of changes in lung function or increasing blood pressure.
   (b) Evaluation of specific symptoms. You will soon learn by working with your physician when symptoms are important and when they represent only transient changes in your physiological or nervous makeup.
   (c) Genetic counseling and long-range planning.

3. Develop a physical conditioning program that will:
   (a) Reduce the resting pulse rate to less than 65.
   (b) Condition the heart to a point where the heart rate can be returned to 100 or less within 10 minutes following 30 minutes of strenuous exercise.
   (c) Increase the vital capacity.
   (d) Increase your energy level and "zest for living."

4. Actively participate in safety procedures and insist on safety for those around you.

It is always preferable to give positive advice. In the previous statements we have told you things to do, relationships that you can establish, and attitudes that you can develop that are important in the quantity and quality of life. I very much dislike telling you that there are some things you cannot do or that you must stop doing. Unfortunately, if we are to reduce mortality and improve the quality of life, there are some things that you must not do. Therefore, the second list is to be headed with the following statement.

Unfortunately you must:

1. Stop smoking.

2. Cut alcohol consumption by at least 50 per cent and preferably 75 per cent.

3. Select your foods so that your serum cholesterol level will be below 175 at all times.

4. Control your caloric intake so that obesity is avoided.

5. Avoid pregnancy under the age of 20 and over the age of 35.

There are the rules. They are the rules, not only to prevent you from being a mortality statistic, but to help you maintain your good health. Good health cannot be purchased at a drug store or any other place of business. You can get some helpful advice from your physician, from your government, and from many other sources, but the maintenance of health is primarily an active, aggressive policy on the part of the individual. No one will give you good health. You cannot inherit good health. It is true that, without healthy ancestors, it is difficult for you to achieve health and longevity. Regardless of his ancestry, each individual must earn his own right to a long and happy life.

There is little need for us to review each of the rules we have listed. After reading the book, it must be apparent to you where each of these rules enters into the program of life preservation. There is one exception. The first rule of the first list deserves some additional elaboration. We emphasized the importance of an attitude of self-preservation in the growing child. We also commented on risk factors at various times; many of the risks are voluntary.

If someone could invent a pill that would keep people from taking needless risks, mankind would be forever in that inventor's debt. I recently read a book by Richard E. Carney entitled *Risk-taking Behavior,* thinking I might discover why people insist on taking risks. This book was stimulating, but I still do not know, nor can I understand, why people take some risks. I accept the fact that children must take risks in order to expand and grow. Many times the child does not realize that he is taking a risk; he is only trying to expand his horizons. This must, in most instances, be considered a worthy risk. When the risk is dangerous to the child, the parent must intervene, and this is referred to as discipline. Adolescents go through the same type of growth by experiment. Of course, man could never have gone to the moon had he not been willing to take risks. It is therefore apparent that risk must be balanced against the factors that lead to growth and learning. These are not the foolish risks that cause me concern.

I am not sure where foolish risks have their origin. Psychiatrists speak of a self-destructive urge that is present in everyone. This may indeed be very important in our need to take risks. There seems to be little doubt that taking risks is important to some persons' egos. The hot-rod driver on our city streets darting in and out of traffic will save himself very little time, but certainly he attracts attention, and this activity apparently satisfies some peculiar need in his ego.

Our line of reasoning in this first rule is that you recognize risks for what they are. If you must take risks, select risks that do not endanger your life and health. It is possible to select risks that may actually be advantageous. For example, enroll in a college course (assuming you are and have been out of school for some time) and run the risk of failure. The embarrassment of a poor or an incomplete grade is a definite risk, but there are some very positive factors should you succeed. The same type of risk exists with our physical fitness suggestions. There is a possibility of harming yourself with a physical fitness program if your approach is not a careful one. However, the rewards from such a program are so great that they more than justify the risk. Financial risks are taken by all of us many times in our lives, but there is invariably the opportunity for success that is disproportionate to the risk.

These types of risks can be just as ego-stimulating as those that produce physical harm: recklessness, overeating, overdrinking, and smoking. These suggested risks do not appeal to our self-destructive impulses, which is the very point I wish to make. It is important to develop the attitude of self-preservation and develop your attitude toward risks and risk-taking to one of growth and development rather than self-destruction.

There is a second component to our first rule, and this relates to one's self-image. I have used the term "an attitude of relaxed confidence." In a book that has dealt almost exclusively with facts and statistics, such a philosophical or psychological heading may seem out of place; however, its importance is beyond my statistical or quantitative ability. In our section dealing with heart disease, we mentioned that most emotions such as fear, anger, and hate result in stimulation to the adrenal glands and release of adrenalin in the circulation.

This not only results in an increase of heart rate, but also tends to produce localized damage to the heart muscle. Long-standing anxiety and insecurity apparently can mediate their effects in a similar manner and most certainly produce a significant deleterious effect over the years. In addition to heart damage, chronic anxieties and chronic stresses reflect themselves in other physiological ways. Such disorders as asthma, peptic ulcer, irritable colon, migraine headaches, and sinus troubles are all aggravated by, or may in some instances actually be produced by, chronic stress and frustration. A very important facet of preventive medicine is, therefore, one of attitude. Every person needs to know and appreciate his own ability; this results in a sense of identity. Also we need to know our own limitations and avoid putting ourselves in situations that are frustrating and impossible. Some persons apparently must experience a myocardial infarction before they can learn that some office responsibilities can be delegated. Some people apparently must be injured in automobile accidents before they learn that they were really not in a great hurry. It is our hope that such lessons can be learned in an easier manner. Take a long look at your station in life, at your job, and how you spend your time, and see where you are comfortable and where you are not comfortable. I know of no magic formula to tell you what you should or should not do, but the answers are very likely stored in your own computer. Those things you enjoy, you do well. Those things you do, but which produce anxiety, you do because you are forced to do for some other reason. Once you have achieved a comfortable relationship with your environment, you will develop a relaxed confidence.

Rules two and three have been discussed extensively.

You are well aware of their importance. Rule four is a general rule regarding safety. I hope that we have convinced you that safety needs to be considered around your home as well as in your automobile. We hope that your safety consciousness will extend far beyond using seat and shoulder belts. We hope that with your next automobile purchase you will emphasize your interest in safety and act accordingly. This is one message Detroit can understand very well. If people refuse to buy the sleek but unsafe automobile and choose one with safety features, it will not be long before the manufacturers will be competing with each other over safety advances rather than styling trends. We have discussed home safety to a moderate degree; disasters can be prevented in the home. Medicine cabinets must be child-proofed. Waxed floors and slick-sole shoes are an invitation to broken bones in the young and to fatalities in the not so young. All of us can be inventive in the area of safety. It takes no more than a survey of your home or job environment and an instinct for self-preservation.

Our second set of rules is certainly no less important than our first. These rules have also been covered throughout the text. I would call your attention to Chart XXXI in the Appendix and comment that this chart is based on the total mortality figures for smokers and nonsmokers. It takes into account all forms of death. You will note that smokers have two to three times the death rate of nonsmokers during the middle years of life. This chart certainly summarizes the hazards of the tobacco risk. The smoker-prone diseases such as death by myocardial infarction, cancer of the lung, and pulmonary emphysema have such a poor or hopeless medical prognosis that the only hope of reducing their disastrous mortality rates is to prevent the disease. If a person were deliberately to select the diseases with the poorest chances of recovery, he could do no better than use the list of diseases that are virtually the sole property of the smoker.

Pipe and cigar smoking reduces the risk only if the smoke is not inhaled. A cigarette smoker can rarely make this transition and not inhale. Persons who smoke need to inspect their ego demands very seriously and see what there is about this risk that is important to them. The opinion has been expressed that smoking is a form of true drug addiction. Most authors, however, feel that this is not the case and that smoking is purely a habit based on some peculiar ego need.

Our insistance that pregnancy not occur under the age of 20 or over the age of 35 is based on our desire to have quality infants. There is less chance for prematurity in the age group indicated, the babies are more apt to be normal, and the mothers do not run as high a mortality and complication rate as those outside this ideal age range. Reproduction is a special privilege. It should be entered into carefully. Reproductive health must be considered one of our most important assets. Follow all of the rules very carefully, and generations to come will thank you.

XV. Results

The basic premise of this book has been that too many people are dying too soon. We have offered you the rules by which people can live and significantly defer death. In each category it has been apparent to you that there are deaths that could have been deferred or, in many instances, taken completely out of one category and moved into a more desirable one. The most extreme example would be death from prematurity. It would have been much better to prevent death from prematurity and defer it until old age. In 1967 there were 1,851,323 deaths. Of those, 715,161 occurred in people under the age of 65. We made what seemed to be a rash statement early in this book when we contended that 100,000 lives could have been salvaged, not from the total large number, but from those who died under the age of 65. At this point I would like to review the deaths that occurred in just nine general categories and see how we think our rules for death deferrment might alter the number of deaths in that year. Let us assume that we are immediately applying our rules to everyone. Let us assume that the death rate for 1967 will be the same, which will serve as a numerical working base. I, of course, understand that the number of deaths per year will increase as the population increases but, in order to make some sense of our figures, let me make the assumption that the number of people who died of disease in 1967 will be the same number that will occur in any subsequent year unless we can do something to improve or reduce the number of deaths in that category. I am also sure that you understand that some of our rules will not produce complete reversal in the mortality figures at any time. Some of these rules must be in effect a number of years before any change in the death rate will be noticed. Therefore, in an attempt to be fair, I am listing in separate columns the deaths that can be deferred next year, the deaths that can be deferred five years from now, and the deaths that can be deferred 15 years from now. Chart XXVII on page 293 lists each category and the numbers indicated. We will discuss each group separately.

Coronary and degenerative heart disease, the first entry on our list, the biggest killer in 1967, has held that infamous but lofty position for a number of years and appears to be firmly entrenched. I, and many of my colleagues are convinced that this is largely a preventable disease. Unfortunately, its prevention cannot be accomplished by immunizing our children. It is also unfortunate that, if all of us changed our ways completely tomorrow, the disease would not instantaneously disappear. I hope that I have given you enough insight into the disease and into the heart and and its physiology to make these statements reasonable. I believe that, if all of us started following the rules we listed in the previous section, there would be a significant decrease in the number of coronary deaths next year. This improvement would come about through the reduction in the number of sudden deaths related to smoking and sedentary living. The reduction in the number of deaths occurring after myocardial infarction should be secondary to the improved collateral circulation and the reduced irritability of the heart muscle that have resulted from discontinuing cigarettes and our physical conditioning program.

Professor A. Fingerland of Czechoslovakia feels that at least half of the deaths caused by myocardial infarction are

Chart XXVII

	TOTAL DEATHS 1967	UNDER AGE 65 - 1967	SAVE NEXT YEAR	SAVE 5 YRS. FROM NOW	SAVE 15 YRS. FROM NOW
ALL CAUSES	1,851,323	715,161			
HEART DISEASE	625,850	167,495	40,000	80,000	100,000
Coronary & Degenerative					
CANCER (total)	310,983	137,967	20,000	30,000	50,000
Lung Cancer	54,407	27,759	---	1,000	20,000
STROKES	202,184	36,761	3,000	6,000	10,000
ACCIDENTS & (Poisons)	60,309	39,041	8,000	10,000	12,000
MOTOR VEHICLE	52,924	45,447	15,000	25,000	30,000
Total Accidents	113,233				
LUNG DISEASE	97,725	34,721			
EMPHYSEMA & Bronchitis	26,181	6,603	500	2,000	5,000
Infectious	71,544	28,118	3,000	4,000	5,000
PREMATURITY	40,253	40,253	8,000	20,000	20,000
CIRRHOSIS OF LIVER	27,816	21,114	500	10,000	15,000
SUICIDE	21,325	17,492	2,000	4,000	6,000
HOMICIDE	13,425	12,672	2,000	2,000	2,000
			102,000	194,000	275,000

intimately associated with cigarette smoking. This is consistent with our data that show that sudden death accounts for at least half of the coronary mortality and that at least 80 per cent of the victims of sudden death are smokers. It is in the area of myocardial infarction that the smoker pays his dues. Despite the association of cancer of the lung and smoking in the public mind, the smoker's risk of being a sudden death heart fatality is at least four times greater than his risk of developing cancer of the lung. Since not all smokers with myocardial infarction die suddenly, an accurate overall estimate of his increased risk is difficult to determine, but there is no doubt that the risk is much greater than that of developing cancer of the lung.

We do know that persons who stop smoking very shortly enjoy reduced myocardial infarction risks. Even after 90 days as a nonsmoker, the heart attack mortality rate is reduced. After one year of nonsmoking the risk is reduced to less than half that of a smoker; each year the risk decreases further. It is difficult to know exactly when the ex-smoker's risk becomes the same as that of a nonsmoker, but in the area of myocardial infarction it seems to be approximately five years. I would hope there would be fewer myocardial infarctions based on physical fitness programs; scientific evidence is beginning to confirm this. We are assuming that persons who have hypertension will be seen by their physicians and begin therapy. Persons who have a high blood cholesterol will be started on diets and other corrective measures. With a combination of these risk corrections, we feel that as much as a 25 per cent reduction in the mortality figures the following year is a conservative estimate. The longer these risk control measures are in effect, the more lives will be saved.

The dietary aspects of myocardial infarction have been discussed in scattered sections of the book. The importance of starting diets directed toward the reduction of arteriosclerosis early in life is again emphasized. Childhood is where it all begins. By emphasizing this fact here, I hope that those parents who do nothing for themselves will at least do something for their children. Mothers, please, stop killing your children with rich foods! Fat babies and fat children are not healthy babies and children. Feed them well, but feed them properly. I sincerely believe that the number of deaths that can be deferred by this practice have been underestimated on this chart.

We have listed cancer of the lung separately from the total entry of cancer. This was done to emphasize the possibilities of preventing cancer of the lung. You will note that 27,759 persons under the age of 65 died of cancer of the lung. We have estimated that, with all of our rules for deferring death, we could not eliminate a single death next year from this cause. Cancer of the lung is a smoker's disease; unfortunately, the changes that result in the lung from smoking are not as quickly reversed as those in the heart. A fair estimate is that aften ten years as an ex-smoker, the incidence of cancer of the lung is only twice as great as it is in the nonsmoker; after perhaps 18 years as an ex-smoker, a person enjoys the same low incidence of cancer of the lung as the nonsmoker.

We have indicated that a number of lives can be saved in the general category of cancer. The estimate of 20,000 lives is conservative compared to the American Cancer Society's estimate of 100,000. I admit that I am more pessimistic about this disease than that organization. We find this disease unpredictable. Early diagnosis is important, and with early diagnosis there is no doubt that some additional lives can be saved. There is also evidence to show that more forms of cancer may be preventable. The virus etiology is extremely exciting and may open a number of new frontiers from which to attack this disease. The number of deaths that can be deferred with cancer control is significant. The number I have given here I believe to be realistic. The American Cancer Society would give you a number virtually three times as great as I have listed. I believe that they are overly optimistic. By all means learn the seven danger signals of cancer (see Chart XXXVII in the Appendix) as published by the American Cancer Society and, above all, avoid fear and despair if you should personally be involved in fighting this disease.

Strokes involve persons primarily over the age of 65. However, 36,761 deaths under age 65 represent a total that should not be ignored. If one is to use a conservative figure and estimate that half of these are related to hypertension, we have a basis on which we can hope for prevention of strokes in the younger age group. This same hope would apply to elderly patients, and in fact, is more advantageous to the patient past 65. Some of the strokes that occur in the younger age groups are related to anomalies of the blood vessels going to the brain, to accidents, or to acute hypertensive episodes that are difficult to control. Greater numbers of strokes are related to more conventional hypertension. We do know that, by reducing the risk factors related to arteriosclerosis and heart disease, there should be a reduction in cerebral vascular disease, as well. The estimate that 9 to 10 per cent of the strokes that kill people under the age of 65 are preventable, I regard as realistic. I would also consider that, if we adopt proper rules of health, the number of deaths that can be deferred from this entity will increase.

I am certain that, if anyone is to criticize my estimates for deaths that could be deferred, that criticism could be launched against this category. I have very probably underestimated the number of lives that could be saved in the accident area. Theoretically, reducing alcohol consumption as indicated in our rules could cut the automobile death rate in half. There is no question that the addition of shoulder harnesses to our lap belts will make for further reductions in the accident mortality. Reduced speed, which is now the law, will also be an important factor. Home accidents involving children are indefensibly high; if the proper attitudes can be developed as we have outlined them in our rules for death deferment, major changes could be made in this category. Eighteen hundred deaths annually from fire caused by careless smoking could be eliminated immediately. However, I fear that the need for self-destruction and what seems to be an inherent carelessness exists in people as they drive automobiles, and this will not be corrected in the foreseeable future. Proper attitudes can be acquired within a generation, and I believe manufacturers of vehicles will be with us once they can be convinced that safety is the paramount feature. Real improvement in this category can occur, but realistically all of us would be appreciative if we could immediately benefit from the gains I have listed.

The category of lung disease does not include cancer of the lung or pneumonia of the newborn. It is divided into two general categories: emphysema and bronchitis, and infectious disease of the lung or pneumonia. Although emphysema and bronchitis take their biggest toll in the age group over 65, they nevertheless took the lives of 6603 persons under the age of 65. Compared to our other categories, this is relatively small. Most patients have 5 to 10 years of significant disability before they succumb to emphysema and bronchitis. Deferring death from this disorder is much the same as deferring death from cancer of the lung. However, if patients with emphysema and bronchitis can be weaned from cigarettes, medical therapy is that much more effective. My colleagues in chest medicine tell me that, unless they can break the cigarette habit, medical therapy in emphysema and bronchitis will achieve only limited success. We feel that these diseases are at least 90 per cent preventable over a 15-to-20-year period. It is on this basis that we have shown a progressive increase in the number of deaths that are deferrable.

Infectious disease of the respiratory tract should be successfully treated with antibiotics. On the basis of that statement, you may wonder why so few deaths are listed in the death-deferrable category over the next 15 years. There is no doubt that pneumonia is a terminal event for many of our very elderly and our very young patients. When the host has lost his resistance to infection, even antibiotics are of limited value. While we can make some improvement in our mortality statistics in infection, it will always be a major killer. As you can see, I have listed an improvement of only approximately 20 per cent over the next 15 years. All physicians would be pleased if this could be accomplished.

The major category of death in the infant period is listed as "certain diseases of early infancy." In 1967 these diseases took 48,314 lives. Prematurity predisposed or actually produced 40,253 of those deaths. I have elected to present only prematurity on our chart of diseases that may represent a significant opportunity for salvage. The medical attack on prematurity has been less than an all-out effort. In addition to this, the public has generally held the attitude that all married females should reproduce. More emphasis has been placed on the morality of reproduction than on the health of the product produced. This area, like accidents, holds tremendous potential for death reduction. Never in history have we been so blessed with safe available birth control measures as we are today. Never in history have we been so fortunate with regard to a liberal attitude that makes it possible for a female actually to choose whether she will become pregnant. This simply means that if, for reasons of health or potentially transmittable disease a woman elects not to have children, she will not be subjected to the criticism that might have befallen her grandmother. We are gradually evolving to some type of sound reasoning in the area of human reproduction. At the moment our nation is experiencing wholesale abortion, even to the point where there is a shortage of quality adoptable infants. With a little more time and social evolution, we will reach a point where some healthy illegitimate children can be delivered and raised by parents who, at this moment, are bearing potentially or predictably handicapped infants.

The high incidence of prematurity that occurs in certain groups has led us to believe that, with moderate foresight, significant reduction in prematurity can be achieved. The premature rate is too high in the young mother, in the diabetic, and in the low socioeconomic groups. All of these categories present conditions that can be corrected. The one exception, of course, is diabetes. Socioeconomic standards are improving. We are now giving concrete help to youngsters in the ghetto. There is no doubt that their nutrition is better than the nutrition of their parents. If the problem of prematurity is to be given consideration by the public, especially by that portion that is female and considering reproduction, the modest measures we have suggested in this text should minimize the number of premature infants. Since gestation requires nine months, it is difficult to produce a large number of corrections in the next year. Even so, I have estimated that there could be 8000 fewer deaths caused by prematurity in the next year. Part of this assumption is based on the fact that physicians are doing a better job of taking care of prematures. I doubt that we can prevent that many premature infants from being born next year; I do think that we can, by simple health measures, prevent probably half that number; the other 4000 I am expecting my neonatologist colleagues to salvage. Five years from now, as a result of serious consideration on the part of the young mothers, and in consequence of the improved nutrition of our younger generation, I feel that nearly half of our current prematures could be born as full-term infants.

Cirrhosis of the liver was the seventh leading cause of death in 1967. Its role as a killer in the American society is increasing. Not all deaths from cirrhosis can be prevented; some are not caused by alcoholism. However, our own experience in this country during prohibition and the current experience of the British, imply that, if alcohol consumption can be reduced by 50 per cent, the death rate will be reduced to one third or one fourth of its present level within four years. If we had some way of knowing which persons were susceptible to alcohol, we might be more selective in indicating who needs to reduce his alcoholic consumption. The most effective way to reduce the alcoholic consumption of the nation by 50 per cent is for every individual to do exactly that. If you drink no alcohol now, you can very easily cut this in half and still drink no alcohol and be perfectly happy. If you drink only at cocktail parties and have two or three drinks at such affairs, simply cut the figure in half. If alcohol is a problem to you or to members of your family, seek professional advice. It may be important for reasons other than preventing cirrhosis to reduce consumption to zero.

Since it requires approximately a four-year lead time in correcting drinking habits before there is any change in the mortality statistics from cirrhosis, we have indicated only a slight reduction in deaths from this cause next year, but have shown progressive improvement over the next 15 years. We are really stating that most cases of cirrhosis of the liver can be prevented.

There are times when suicide represents a successful escape from an impossible situation. In such a case, I do not feel suicide should be prevented. Our society has been too critical of suicide. It is difficult to understand why such an attitude exists. Suicide occurs either in the group that finds an escape or to the person who is too ill to be responsible for making the proper decisions. I see nothing morally involved in either case. It is important that we identify the patient who is sick emotionally and contemplating suicide and make every effort to correct that illness. Suicide in the depressed patient and in the adolescent is a true disaster. If it can be prevented, the underlying problem can be corrected or in time it corrects itself, and the person has many productive years ahead. The identification of potential suicide patients is an extremely important procedure. All of us must have friends and all of us must be concerned about our friends. When suicidal traits appear, we must get these people into the hands of those with specialized skill in treating this emotional disorder. The cure rate in many of our psychological diseases, including alcoholism, is still considerably better than the cure rate for many malignant diseases.

Homicides can be prevented only by attitudes. I would hope that our attitudes toward self-preservation and self-reassurance would be sufficient to stop homicide. Certainly, if the proper attitudes could be instilled in the total population, homicide would not occur. Homicides are predominantly the product of fits of passion; anger and frustration are their parents. Gun laws would probably help reduce the number of homicides, but certainly would not eliminate them. As you can see, virtually all homicides occur under the age of 65. I am most concerned with the homicides involving children, as these are so often perpetrated by a sick parent or parent figure. In this case, the homicide victim is entirely innocent, and society loses what might be a long productive life. The validity of mortality statistics can be challenged in every category, but certainly homicide in infants is underdiagnosed. Our greatest hope is that, with improved attitudes toward having and rearing children, homicide in this age group will disappear. Because homicides are difficult to control and predict, we have listed only 2000 deferrable deaths from this cause. If our government would enact stricter gun laws, even more deferrable deaths in this category might be achieved.

There are the totals: 102,000 deaths deferred next year, 194,000 deferred 5 years from now, and 280,000 deaths deferred 15 years from now. I believe these are very realistic figures. We can attain these figures with a system that requires only self-discipline. At no place in this book have we asked you to contribute large sums of money to anyone or anything. You have the power to do everything that has been suggested here, and you have the power to do so now. It is health power. You need not wait for additional research. Improvement in our environment through ecological efforts would be helpful, but we have not insisted that this be a prerequisite to any of the statistics offered here. We are a rich and wasteful nation. Our waste and pillage of our natural resources do us little credit. However, very little has been said or done about the greatest waste of all. I have devoted this entire text to presenting that waste to you. There is no waste greater and none more significant than the waste of human life. It is truly up to you—you can stay healthy and alive. You can reap the rewards of your life style.

No matter what your age, you're *too young to die!*

Appendix

Chart I

MORTALITY FROM 15 LEADING CAUSES OF DEATH: UNITED STATES, 1967*

Rank order	Cause of Death	Rate	Percent of total deaths
	All Causes	935.7	100.0
1	Diseases of heart	364.5	39.0
2	Malignant neoplasms, including neoplasms of lymphatic and hematopoietic	157.2	16.8
3	Vascular lesions affecting central nervous system	102.2	10.9
4	Accidents	57.2	6.1
--	Motor vehicle accidents	26.7	2.9
--	Other accidents	30.4	3.2
5	Influenza and pneumonia, except pneumonia of newborn	28.8	3.1
6	Certain diseases of early infancy	24.4	2.6
7	General arteriosclerosis	19.0	2.0
8	Diabetes mellitus	17.7	1.9
9	Other diseases of circulatory system	15.1	1.6
10	Other bronchopulmonic disease	14.8	1.6
11	Cirrhosis of liver	14.1	1.6
12	Suicide	10.8	1.5
13	Congenital malformations	8.8	0.9
14	Homicide	6.8	0.7
15	Other hypertensive disease	5.6	0.6
16	All other causes	88.7	9.5

*From U.S. Vital Statistics, Vol. II, 1967.

Chart II

DEATH RATES FOR THE 10 LEADING CAUSES OF DEATH: UNITED STATES, 1971
(Based on a 10-percent sample of deaths. Rates per 100,000 population.)

Rank	Cause of death	Death rate	Percent of total deaths
	All causes	929.0	100.0
1	Diseases of heart	358.4	38.6
2	Malignant neoplasms, including neoplasms of lymphatic and hematopoietic tissue	160.9	17.3
3	Cerebrovascular diseases	100.6	10.8
4	Accidents	53.8	5.8
5	Influenza and pneumonia	27.2	2.9
6	Certain causes of mortality in early infancy	19.2	2.1
7	Diabetes mellitus	18.2	2.0
8	Cirrhosis of liver	15.5	1.7
9	Arteriosclerosis	15.5	1.7
10	Bronchitis, emphysema and asthma	14.5	1.6
--	All other causes	145.3	15.6

Chart III

DEATH RATE PER 100,000

Age	Number
Under 1 year	2,233.1
1-4 Years	86.3
5-9 Years	42.1
10-14 Years	40.7
15-19 Years	102.7
20-24 Years	134.1
25-29 Years	136.8
30-34 Years	169.7
35-39 Years	246.7
40-44 Years	370.2
45-49 Years	577.6
50-54 Years	898.6
55-59 Years	1,374.8
60-64 Years	2,028.1
65-69 Years	3,070.5
70-74 Years	4,603.1
75-79 Years	6,619.6
80-84 Years	10,144.3
85 & Above	19,419.7

*Derived from U.S. Vital Statistics, 1967.

Chart IV

EXPECTATION OF LIFE IN ANCIENT AND MODERN TIMES

(ANCIENT ROME COMPARED WITH UNITED STATES)

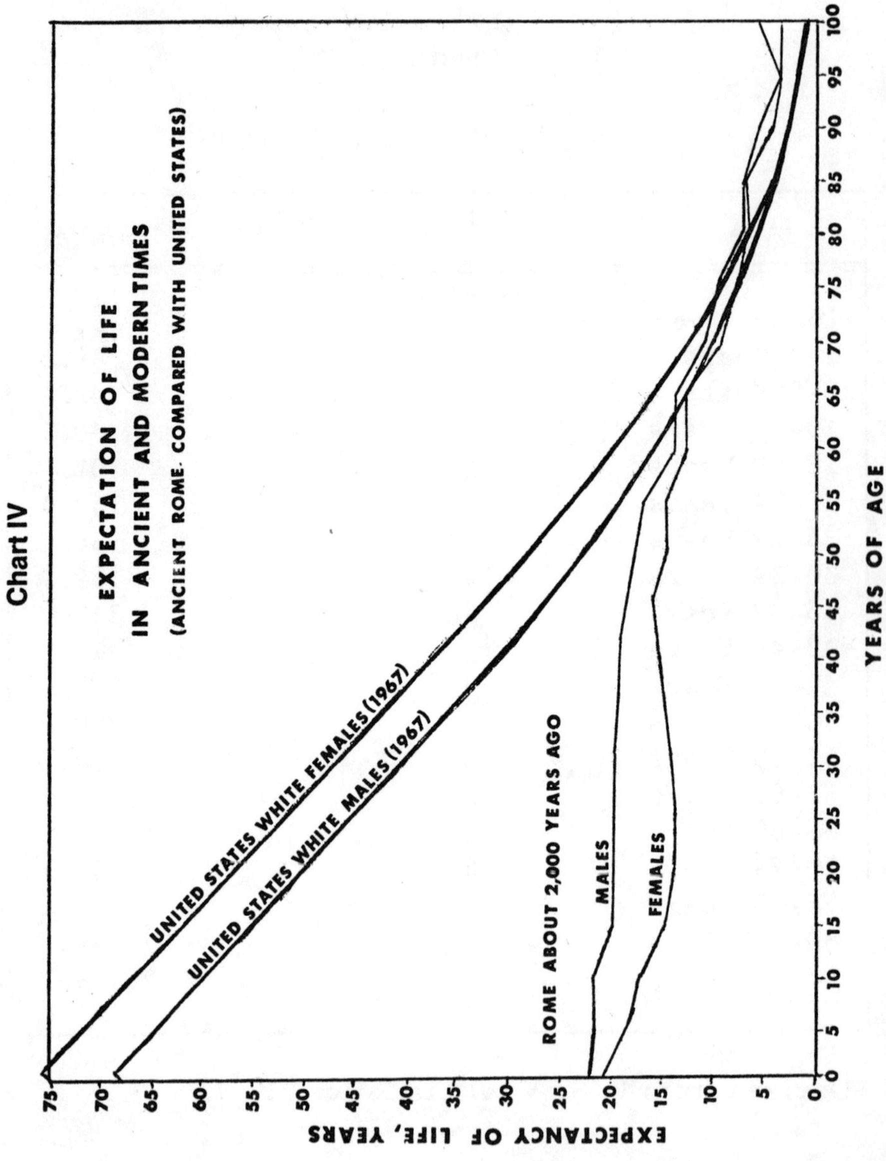

Chart V

MORTALITY
FIRST TWENTY-EIGHT DAYS OF LIFE

Cause of Death	Number
1. Congenital Anomalies	8,342
2. Certain Diseases of Newborn	47,382
Prematurity playing important role in	39,354
3. Infections (Other than 2)	1,419
4. Accidents	311
5. Homicides	117
6. Malignancy	37
7. Other	519
TOTAL	58,127

*Derived from U.S. Vital Statistics 1967.

Chart VI

CERTAIN DISEASES OF NEWBORN

Birth Injuries
Post-natal Asphyxia & Atelectasis
Pneumonia of Newborn
Diarrhea of Newborn
Other Infections of Newborn

(Neonatal Disorders Arising From Maternal Disorders)
Hemolytic Disease of Newborn
Hemorrhagic Disease of Newborn
Nutrition Maladjustments of Newborn
Unqualified Immaturity

Chart VII

ACTUAL NUMBER OF DEATHS
PER MONTH OF LIFE

AGE	NUMBER OF DEATHS
28 - 59 Days	5,277
2 Months	4,012
3 Months	2,903
4 Months	2,095
5 Months	1,617
6 Months	1,325
7 Months	967
8 Months	827
9 Months	685
10 Months	614
11 Months	579

*Derived from U. S. Vital Statistics 1967.

Chart VIII

MORTALITY
TWENTY-EIGHTH DAY TO END OF YEAR ONE

Cause of Death	Number
1. Congenital Anomalies	3,782
2. Certain Diseases of Newborn	889
Prematurity a factor in	303
3. Infection - All Types	10,778
4. Accidents - All Types	2,440
5. Ill Defined Symptoms	1,937
6. Homicides	109
7. Malignancy	159
8. Other	807
TOTAL	20,901

*Derived from U.S. Vital Statistics 1967.

Chart IX

ACCIDENTAL DEATHS
UNDER ONE YEAR OF AGE

Type of Accident	Number
Ingestion of Inhalation of Food or Objects	620
Crib Deaths	522
Motor Vehicle Accidents	321
Fire	189
Falls	163
Drowning	68
Poison with solid, liquid or gas	61
Other	807

*Derived from U.S. Vital Statistics, 1967.

Chart X

IMMUNIZE YOUR CHILD*

Measles, rubella, polio, whooping cough, diphtheria and tetanus are not just harmless childhood diseases. All of them can cripple or kill.

All are preventable. In order to be completely protected against diphtheria, tetanus and whooping cough (pertussis) your child needs a shot of the combination diphtheria-tetanus-pertussis (DTP) vaccine at two, four, six, and eighteen months and a booster when he goes to school.

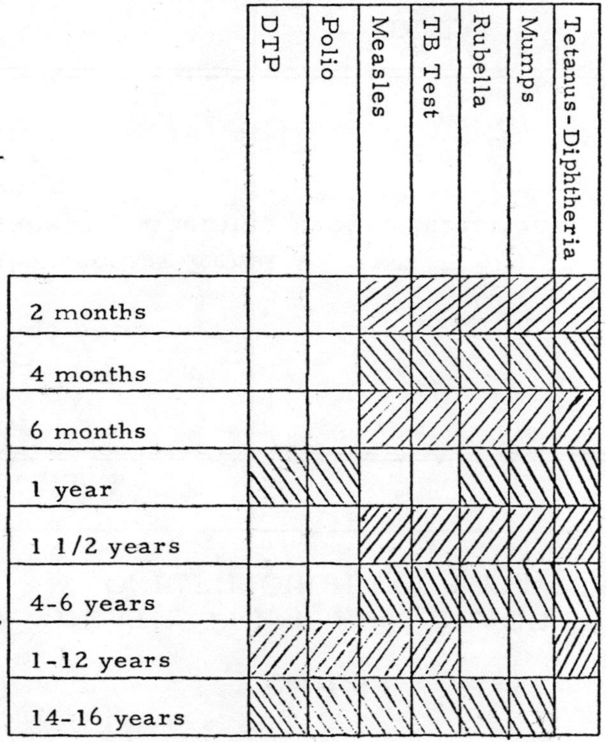

When he gets his DTP shots he should also get a drop of the oral polio vaccine.

After his first birthday your child should have a shot for measles, rubella and mumps. This also can be given in one combination shot. He should be tested for tuberculosis in his first year, and when he's 14 to 16 years make sure he gets his tetanus diphtheria booster shot.

*Recommended by The American Academy of Pediatrics

Published by the American Academy of Pediatrics.

Chart XI

DEATHS PER 100,000 IN AGE GROUP
ONE THROUGH FOUR YEARS*

Cause of Death	Number
1. Accidents	32.4
2. Infections	23.6
3. Congenital Anomalies	9.7
4. Malignancy	8.2
5. Major Cardiovascular Renal	1.9
6. Asthma, Diabetes, Anemia, Ulcer, Intestinal Obstruction	1.8
7. Homicide	1.1
8. Other	7.6
TOTAL	86.3

*Compiled from U.S. Vital Statistics, Vol. II, 1967.

Chart XII

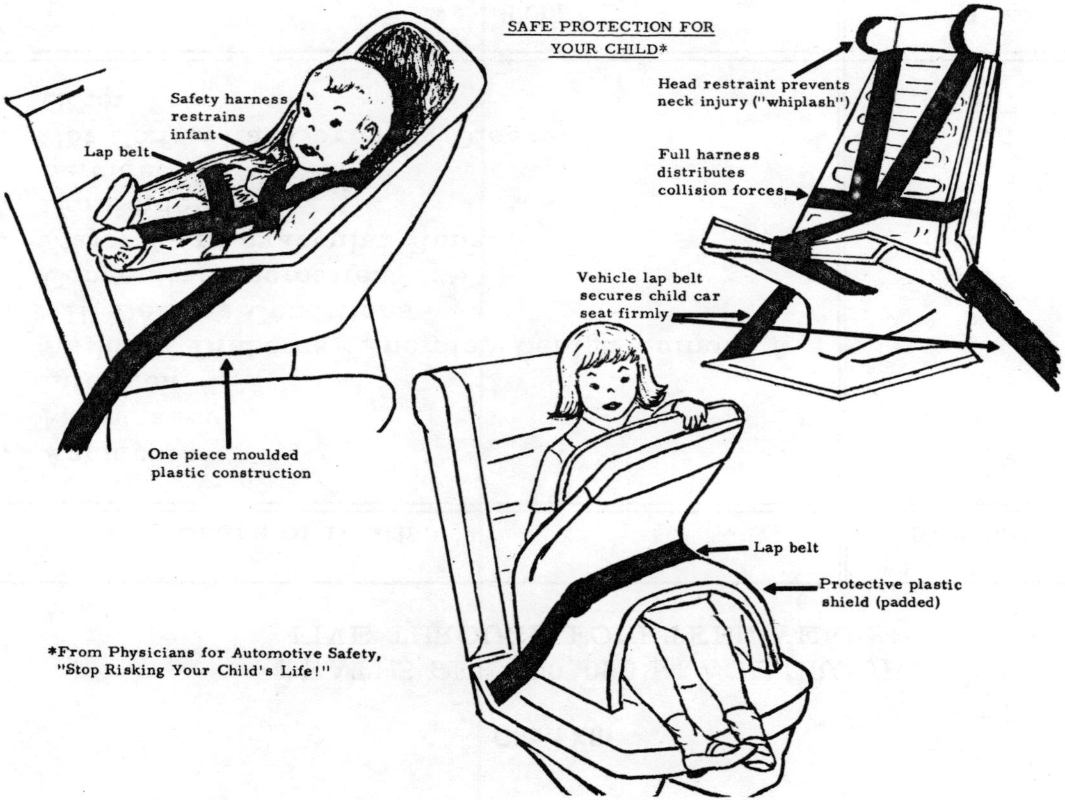

*From Physicians for Automotive Safety, "Stop Risking Your Child's Life!"

Chart XIII

DEATHS PER 100,000 IN AGE GROUP FIVE THROUGH FOURTEEN YEARS*

Cause of Death	Number
1. Accidents	19.3
2. Malignancy	6.6
3. Infection	3.9
4. Asthma, Diabetes, Anemia, Benign Tumors & Ill Defined Conditions	2.6
5. Congenital Anomalies	2.4
6. Major Cardiovascular Renal	1.9
7. Homicide	.7
8. Suicide	.3
9. Not Congenital Coronary Disease	.1
10. Other	3.7
TOTAL	41.4

*Compiled from U.S. Vital Statistics, Vol. II, 1967.

Chart XIV

DEATHS PER 100,000 IN AGE GROUP FIFTEEN THROUGH TWENTY-FOUR YEARS*

Cause of Death	Number
1. Accidents	67.1
2. Homicide	9.1
3. Malignancy	8.3
4. Suicide	7.0
5. Major Cardiovascular Renal	6.5
6. Infection	4.4
7. Asthma, Diabetes, Anemia, Benign Tumors, Ulcer, Intestinal Obstruction & Hernia	2.6
8. Congenital Anomalies	2.2
9. Complication of Pregnancy, Abortion or Child Birth	2.0
10. Other	7.7
TOTAL	116.9

*Compiled from U.S. Vital Statistics, Vol. II, 1967.

Chart XV

DEATHS PER 100,000 IN AGE GROUP
TWENTY-FIVE THROUGH THIRTY-FOUR YEARS*

Cause of Death	Number
1. Accidents	52.0
2. Major Cardiovascular Renal	22.3
3. Malignancy	17.5
4. Homicides	14.6
5. Suicide	12.4
6. Asthma, Diabetes, Anemia, Benign Tumors, Ulcer Intestinal Obstruction, Hernia, Senility, Ill Defined Conditions	8.9
7. Infections	5.8
8. Cirrhosis of Liver	4.0
9. Birth Defects	1.6
10. Complications of Pregnancy, Abortion & Child Birth	1.6
11. Pulmonary Disease other than Pneumonia, Bronchitis or Neoplasia	.5
12. Other	11.2
TOTAL	152.4

Chart XVI

DEATHS PER 100,000 IN AGE GROUP
THIRTY-FIVE THROUGH FORTY-FOUR YEARS*

Cause of Death	Number
1. Major Cardiovascular Renal	98.2
2. Malignancy	60.3
3. Accidents	47.8
4. Cirrhosis of Liver	17.2
5. Infections	16.3
6. Suicide	16.1
7. Asthma, Anemia, Benign Tumors, Ulcer, Intestinal Obstruction, Hernia, Senility, & Ill Defined Symptoms	13.6
8. Homicide	12.1
9. Diabetes	4.8
10. Pulmonary Disease other than Infection or Neoplasia	2.1
11. Birth Defects	1.8
12. Complications of Pregnancy	1.1
13. Other	18.3
TOTAL	310.6

*Compiled from U.S. Vital Statistics, Vol. II, 1967.

Chart XVII

SCHEMATIC DRAWING OF CONDUCTION SYSTEM OF THE HEART

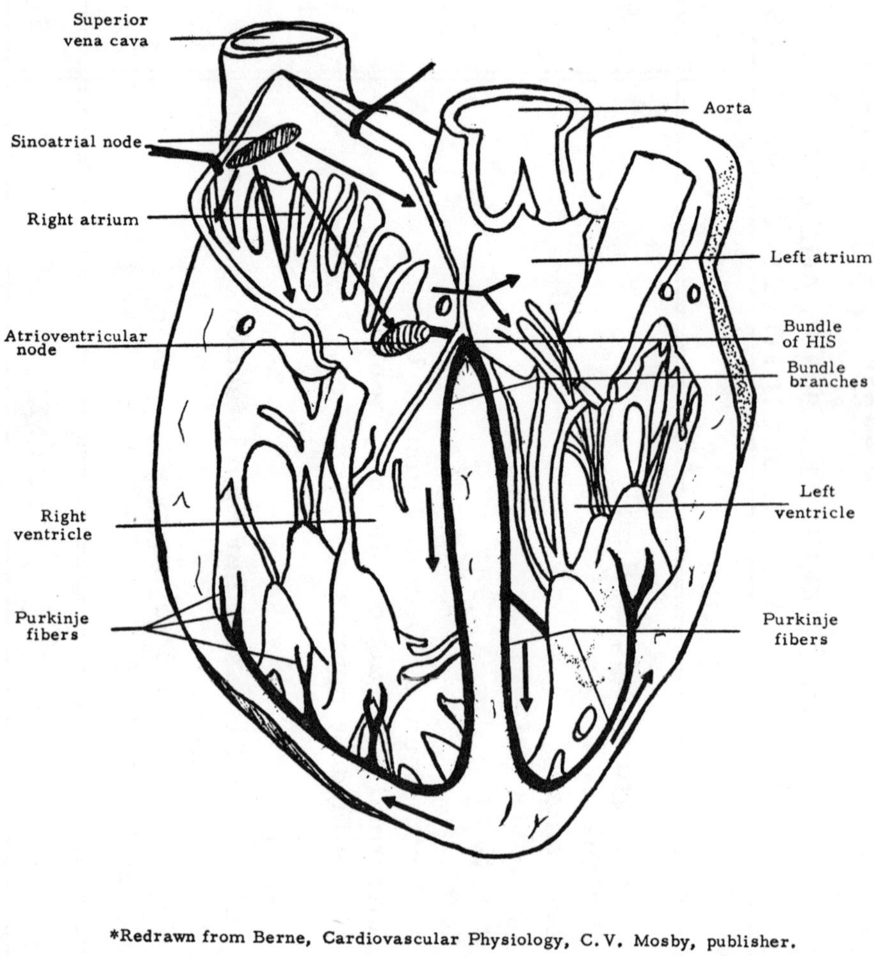

*Redrawn from Berne, Cardiovascular Physiology, C. V. Mosby, publisher.

Chart XVIII

CORONARY ARTERIES OF THE HEART

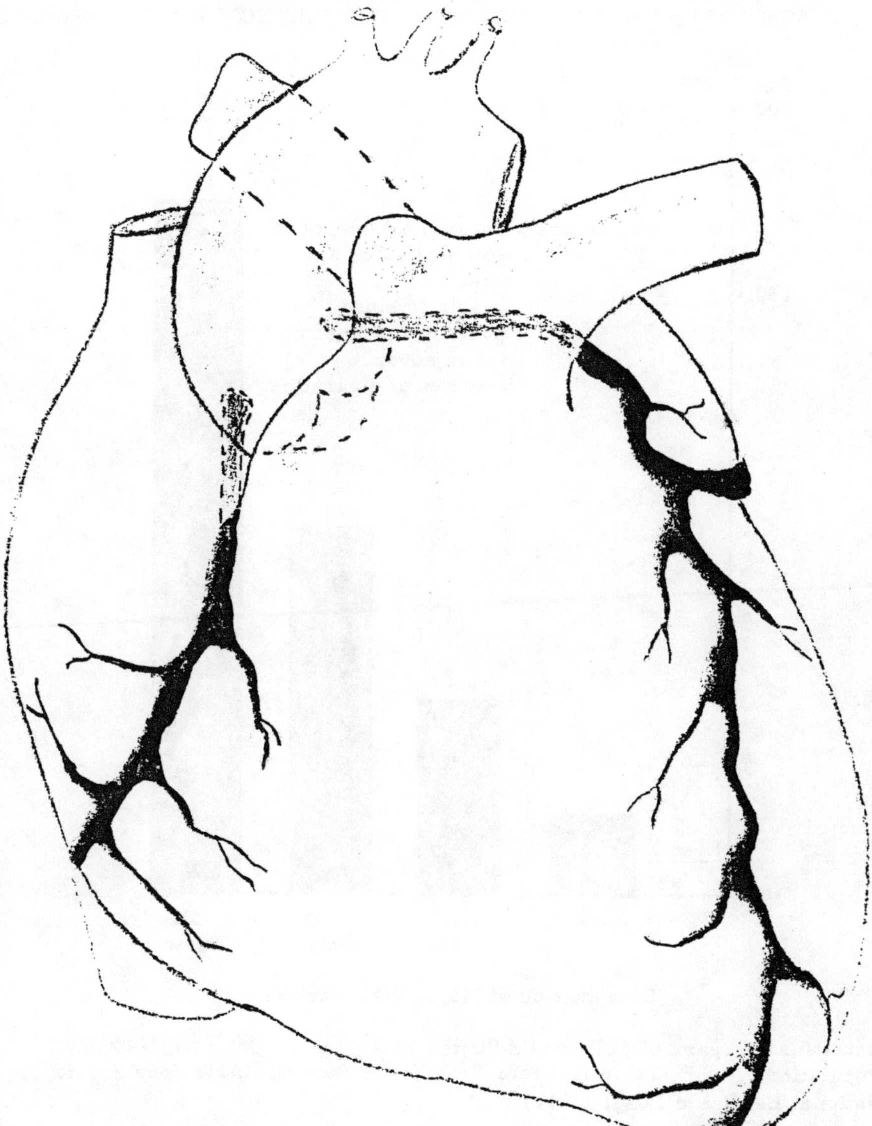

Chart XIX

COMBINATION OF RISK FACTORS AT ENTRY AND AGE-ADJUSTED RATES* OF FIRST MAJOR CORONARY EVENT FOR WHITE MALES AGE 30-59 AT ENTRY. NATIONAL COOPERATIVE POOLING PROJECT

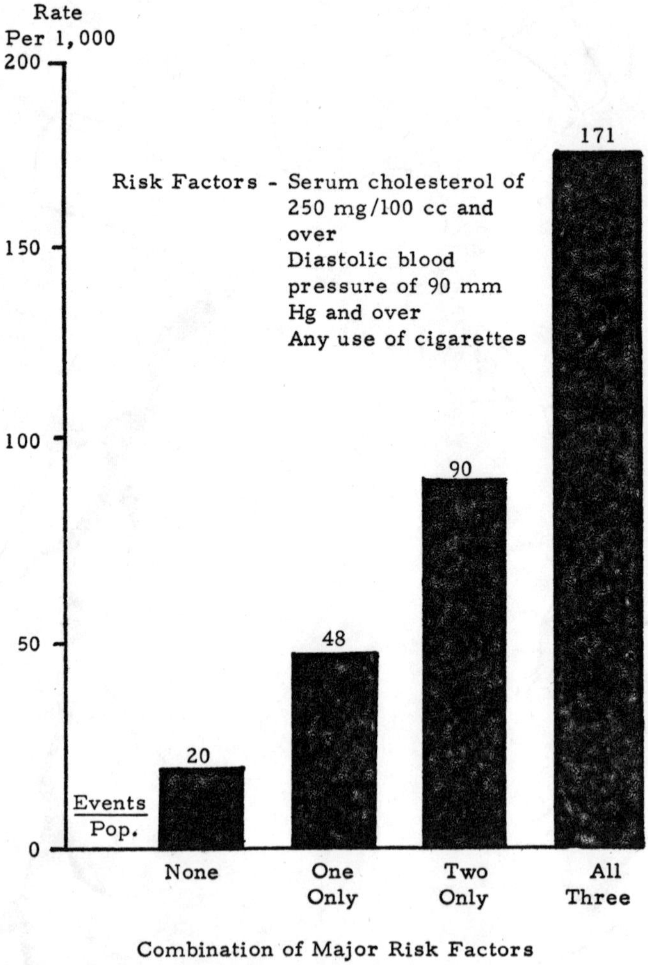

*Rates for 10 Years of Followup Adjusted by Age to the U.S. White Male Population. (From Institute Task Force Report, "Arteriosclerosis", National Heart and Lung, 1971.)

CORONARY HEART DISEASE MORTALITY

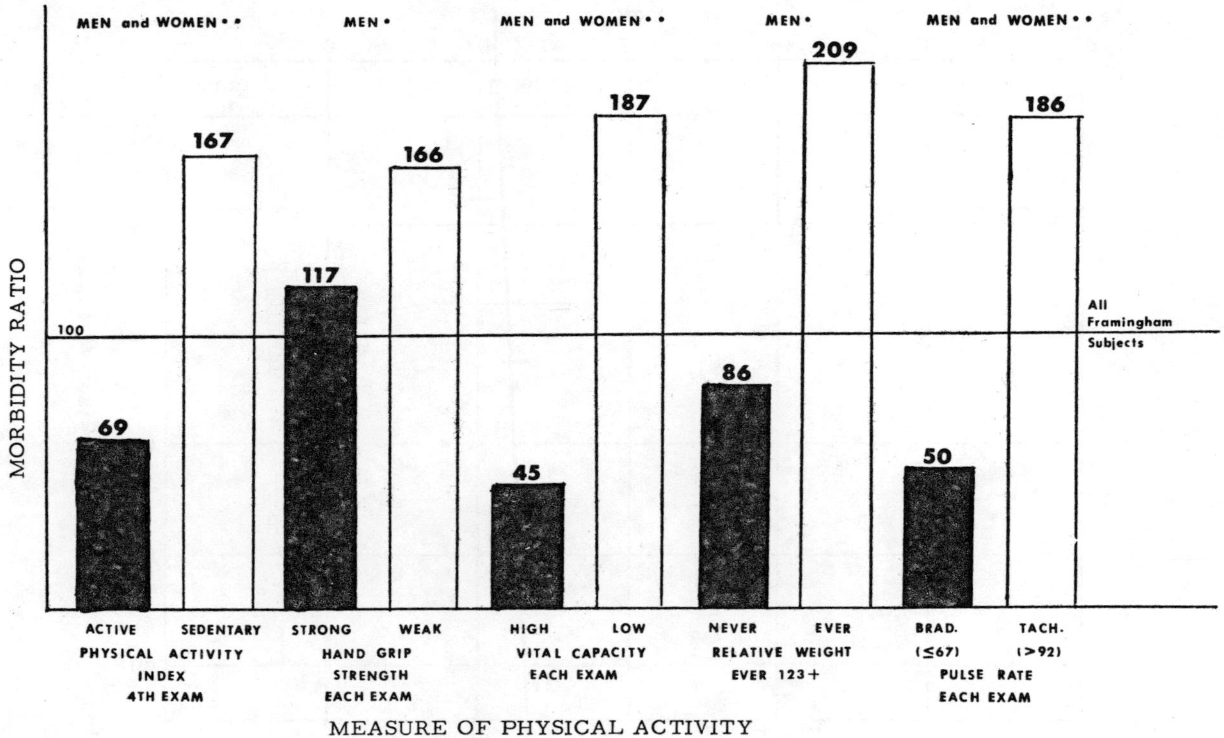

*From the Framingham Heart Study, William B. Kannel, M.D., U.S. Department of Health, Education, and Welfare.

Chart XXI

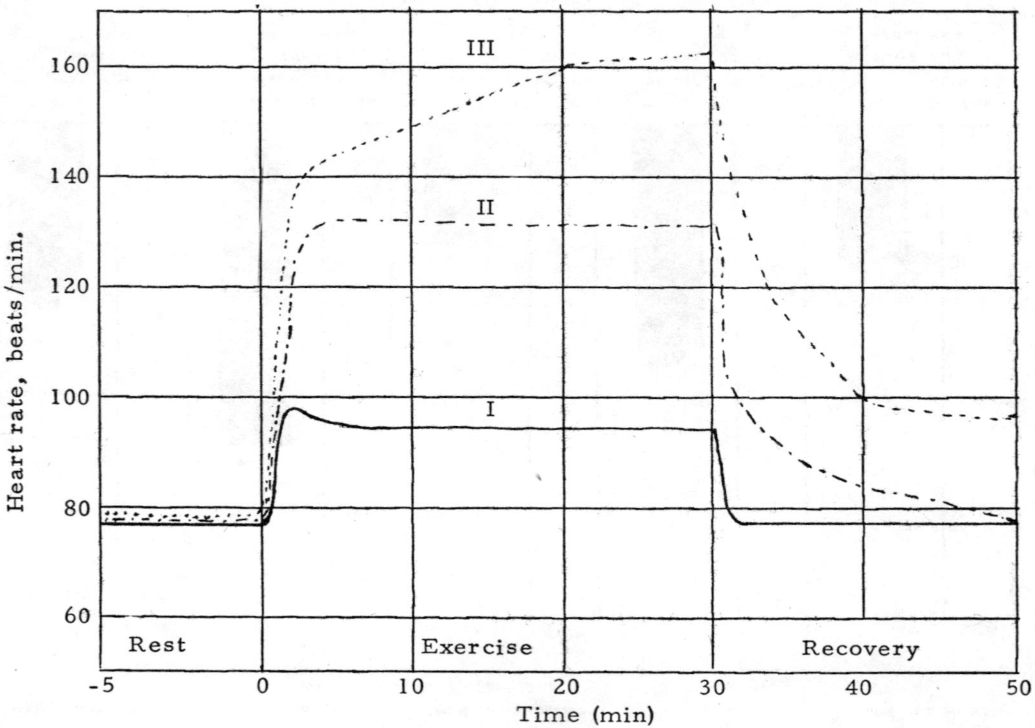

Heart rate response to exercise of different degree. I, light exercise; II, moderate exercise; III, heavy exercise.

Chart XXII

NECESSARY PULSE RATE FOR TRAINING EFFECT

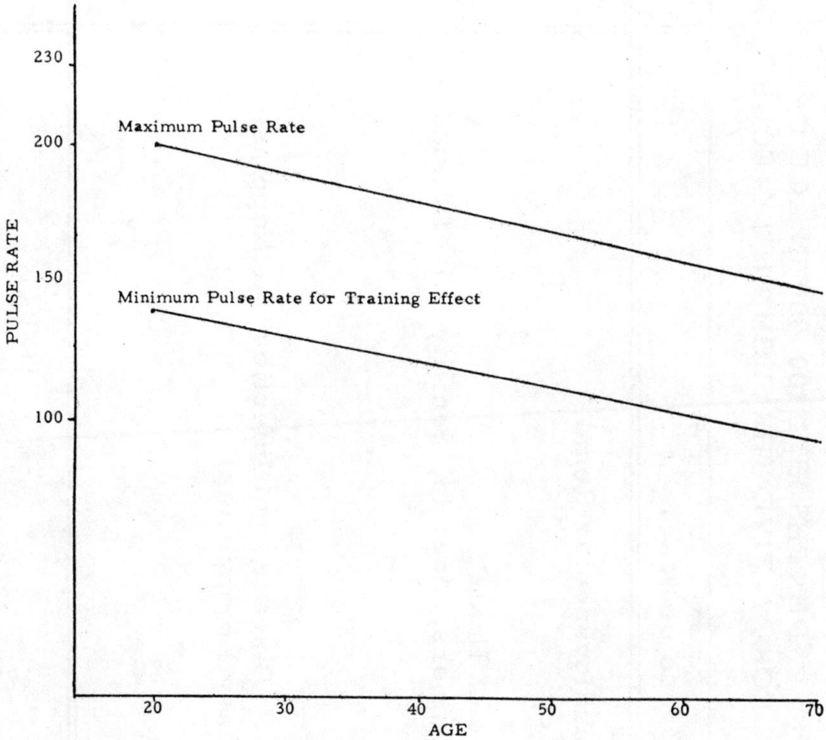

*Derived from data from Raab, W, "Preventive Myocardiology", Chas. Thomas, Publisher, and Fox, S.M., et al, "Physical Activity and the Prevention of Coronary Heart Disease", Annals of Clinical Research 3:404-432, 1971.

Chart XXIII

DEATHS PER 100,000 IN AGE GROUP
FORTY-FIVE THROUGH FIFTY-FOUR YEARS*

Cause of Death	Number
1. Major Cardiovascular Renal	317.9
2. Malignancy	179.4
3. Accidents	54.1
4. Cirrhosis of Liver	34.8
5. Benign Tumors, Anemia, Senility & Ill Defined Symptoms	27.3
6. Infections	23.9
7. Suicide	19.5
8. Diabetes	12.3
9. Pulmonary Diseases not Infectious or Neoplastic (Pulmonary Emphysema)	9.1
10. Homicide	8.2
11. Birth Defects	2.7
12. Other	42.5
TOTAL	730.7

DEATHS PER 100,000 IN AGE GROUP
FIFTY-FIVE THROUGH SIXTY-FOUR YEARS*

Cause of Death	Number
1. Major Cradiovascular Renal	863.7
2. Malignancy	412.4
3. Infections	72.7
4. Accidents	66.0
5. Asthma, Ulcer, Intestinal Obstruction, Benign Tumor, Anemia, Senility	55.0
6. Cirrhosis of Liver	45.7
7. Diabetes	36.2
8. Pulmonary Disease not Infectious or Neoplastic (Pulmonary Emphysema)	35.6
9. Suicide	22.4
10. Homicide	5.6
11. Birth Defects	2.9
12. Other	55.8
TOTAL	1674.0

*Compiled from U.S. Vital Statistics, Vol. II, 1967.

Chart XXV

DEATHS PER 100,000 IN AGE GROUP
SIXTY-FIVE THROUGH SEVENTY-FOUR YEARS*

Cause of Death	Number
1. Major Cardiovascular Renal	2247.5
2. Malignancy	768.8
3. Infections	157.5
4. Emphysema & Bronchitis	102.1
5. Diabetes	94.2
6. Accidents	91.2
7. Cirrhosis of Liver	41.1
8. Suicide	19.8
9. Homicide	4.2
10. Birth Defects	2.8
11. Other	220.7
TOTAL	3749.9

*Compiled from U. S. Vital Statistics, Vol. II, 1967.

Chart XXVI

DEATHS PER 100,000 IN AGE GROUP
SEVENTY-FIVE THROUGH EIGHTY-FOUR YEARS*

Cause of Death	Number
1. Major Cardiovascular Renal	5410.7
2. Malignancy	1102.1
3. Infections	414.8
4. Accidents	189.7
5. Diabetes	169.4
6. Emphysema & Bronchitis	145.9
7. Cirrhosis of Liver	27.4
8. Suicide	21.0
9. Homicide	3.2
10. Birth Defects	3.2
11. Other	412.8
TOTAL	7900.2

* Compiled from U.S. Vital Statistics, Vol. II, 1967.

Chart XXVII

	TOTAL DEATHS 1967	UNDER AGE 65 - 1967	SAVE NEXT YEAR	SAVE 5 YRS. FROM NOW	SAVE 15 YRS. FROM NOW
ALL CAUSES	1,851,323	715,161			
HEART DISEASE Coronary & Degenerative	625,850	167,495	40,000	80,000	100,000
CANCER (total)	310,983	137,967	20,000	30,000	50,000
Lung Cancer	54,407	27,759	---	1,000	20,000
STROKES	202,184	36,761	3,000	6,000	10,000
ACCIDENTS & (Poisons)	60,309	39,041	8,000	10,000	12,000
MOTOR VEHICLE	52,924	45,447	15,000	25,000	30,000
Total Accidents	113,233				
LUNG DISEASE	97,725	34,721			
EMPHYSEMA & Bronchitis	26,181	6,603	500	2,000	5,000
Infectious	71,544	28,118	3,000	4,000	5,000
PREMATURITY	40,253	40,253	8,000	20,000	20,000
CIRRHOSIS OF LIVER	27,816	21,114	500	10,000	15,000
SUICIDE	21,325	17,492	2,000	4,000	6,000
HOMICIDE	13,425	12,672	2,000	2,000	2,000
			102,000	194,000	275,000

Chart XXVIII

MORTALITY RATE
(Ten Year Trends)

Cause of Death	1967	1966	1965	1964	1963	1962	1961	1960	1959	1958
All Causes	935.7	951.3	943.2	939.6	961.3	945.0	929.5	954.7	938.6	950.8
All Malignant Diseases	157.2	155.1	153.5	151.3	151.3	149.9	149.4	149.2	147.3	146.8
Major Cardiovascular-Renal	511.5	521.4	516.4	514.3	527.3	521.2	511.4	521.8	515.9	523.5
Coronary Heart Disease and Seq.	316.3	320.1	316.0	315.8	319.5	313.2	304.2	307.4	300.4	300.0
Hypertension	25.3	27.7	28.4	40.0	32.4	33.4	34.6	37.0	28.6	42.7
Strokes	102.2	104.6	103.7	103.6	106.6	106.2	105.4	108.0	104.4	110.1
Emphysema & Bronchitis	14.8	14.5	13.7	12.2	12.3	10.8	9.7	9.6	8.5	8.2
Tuberculosis	3.5	3.9	4.1	4.3	4.9	5.1	5.4	6.1	6.5	7.1
Renal	5.0	5.3	5.5	5.8	6.0	6.1	6.3	6.7	7.0	8.0
Diabetes	17.7	17.7	17.1	16.9	17.2	16.8	16.4	16.7	15.9	15.9
Cirrhosis of Liver	14.1	13.6	12.8	12.1	11.9	11.7	11.3	11.3	10.9	10.8
Syphilis & Seq.	.3	.3	.3	.3	.4	.4	.4	.4	.5	.5
Deliveries & All Complications	.5	.5	.6	.7	.8	.8	.9	.9	.9	.9
Birth Defects	8.8	9.3	10.1	10.6	11.0	11.4	12.0	12.2	12.3	12.4
Certain Diseases of Infancy	24.4	26.4	28.6	31.5	33.2	34.5	35.9	37.4	38.5	39.8
Suicide	10.8	10.9	11.1	10.8	11.0	10.9	10.4	10.6	10.6	10.7
Homicide	6.8	5.9	5.5	5.1	4.9	4.8	4.7	4.7	4.6	4.5
Accidents	57.2	58.0	55.7	54.3	53.4	52.3	50.4	52.3	52.2	52.3

*From Vital Statistics, General Mortality, Vol. II, 1968.

Chart XXIX

ESTIMATED NUMBER OF ILLEGITIMATE LIVE BIRTHS, BY LIVE-BIRTH ORDER AND COLOR: UNITED STATES, 1967*

Live-birth order	Total	White	Non-white
Total	318,100	142,200	175,800
First child	188,800	98,800	89,900
Second child	53,500	18,500	35,000
Third child	25,900	8,800	17,100
Fourth child	15,800	5,600	10,200
Fifth child and over	30,600	8,000	22,600
Not stated	3,400	2,500	900

NOTE: Due to an error in classifying approximately 20,000 births by live-birth order, the number with birth order not stated is inflated.

*From U.S. Vital Statistics Natality, Vol. 1, 1967.

Chart XXX

HUMAN FETOTOXIC MEDICAMENTS*

Maternal Medication	Fetal or Neonatal Effect
(Established human teratogenic drugs)	
Thalidomide	Fetal death or phocomelia, deafness, cerebrovascular, gastrointestinal or genitourinary anomalies
Sex hormones	Masculinization, advanced bone age
Androgens, progestogens, estrogens	
Antineoplastic agents	Multiple anomalies, abortion
Antimetabolities, amethopterin, 5-fluorouracil (5-FU, DON, 6-azauridine, etc.	
Antibiotics: amphotericin B, mitomycin, etc.	
(Possible human teratogenic drugs)	
Vitamin D	Cardiopathies
Antihistamines	Anomalies (?)
Hallucinogens	"Fractured chromosomes," anomalies (?)
Lysergic acid (LSD), mescaline, etc.	
Antidiabetes drugs	Anomalies (?)
Sulfonylurea derivatives	
Corticosteroids	Cleft palate, harelip (?)
Insulin (shock or hypoglycemia)	Anomalies (?)
Antithyroid drugs	Goiter, mental retardation
Thiouracils, inorganic iodides (potassium iodide, etc)	
(Human fetotoxic agents)	
Analgesics, narcotic drugs	
Heroin, morphine	Neonatal death or convulsions, tremors
Salicylates (excessive)	Neonatal bleeding
Anticoagulant drugs	Fetal death or hemorrhage
The coumarins	
Anti-infective drugs	
Chloramphenicol	Neonatal death ("gray syndrome")
Chloroquine	Death or deafness or retinal hemorrhage
Erythromycin	Hepatic injury
Nitrofurantoin	Hemolytic reactions
Novobiocin	Hyperbilirubinemia
Quinine, quinidine	Nerve deafness, thrombocytopenia
Streptomycin	Nerve deafness
Sulfonamides (Kynex, Medicil)	Kernicterus
Tetracyclines	Hemolysis, hepatotoxicity, inhibition of bone growth, discolored teeth
Cardiovascular drugs	
Ammonium chloride	Acidosis
Hexamethonium	Neonatal ileus
Reserpine	Nasal congestion, drowsiness
Thiazides	Thrombocytopenia
Polio vaccine (Sabin)	Death or neurologic damage
Sedatives, hypnotics, tranquilizers	
Meprobamate	Retarded development
Phenobarbital (excessive)	Neonatal bleeding
Phenothiazines	Hyperbilirubinemia
Smallpox (cowpox) vaccine	Death or fetal vaccinia
Tobacco smoking	Undersized babies
Vitamin K (excessive)	Hyperbilirubinemia

*From Bobson & Benson, Management of High Risk Pregnancy & Intensive Care of the Neonate, C. V. Mosby Company, 1971.

Chart XXXI

DEATH RATE (logarithmic scale) PLOTTED AGAINST AGE,

PROSPECTIVE STUDY OF MORTALITY IN U. S. VETERANS*

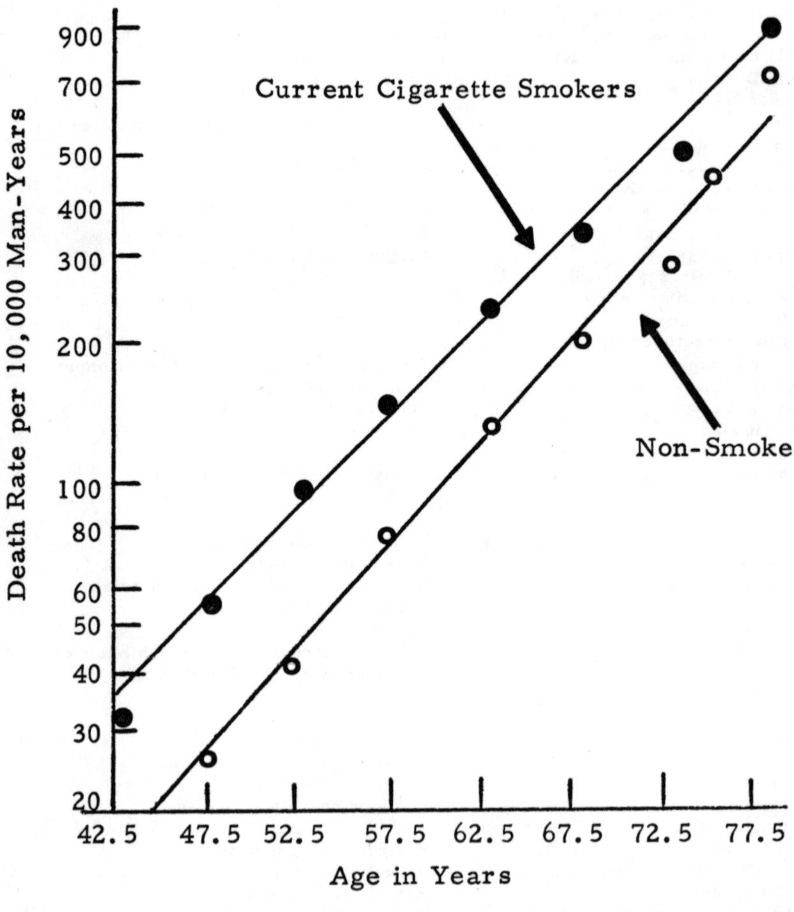

*From Smoking & Health, U.S. Surgeon General 1964.

Chart XXXII

Number of Deaths by Cause of Death and Broad Age Groups

United States, 1967**

Cause of Death	All ages	Under age 65	Age 65 and Over*
All Causes	1,851,323	715,161	1,136,162
Cardiovascular disease (330-334, 400-468)	1,002,111	250,977	751,134
Arteriosclerotic and degenerative heart diseases (420-422)	625,850	167,495	458,355
Vascular lesions affecting central nervous system (330-334)	202,184	36,761	165,423
Diseases of arteries (450-456)	53,326	6,911	46,415
Hypertensive heart disease and hypertension (440-447)	61,126	15,542	45,415
Other diseases of the heart (430-434)	31,267	10,302	20,965
Rheumatic fever and rheumatic heart disease (400-416)	14,176	8,930	5,246
Diseases of the veins and other diseases of the circulatory system (460-468)	14,182	5,036	9,146
Other Causes of Death	849,212	464,184	385,028

*Includes age not stated

Note: Numbers in parenthesis are codes of the International Classification of Diseases, Seventh Revision

** From Institute Task Force Report, "Arteriosclerosis", National Heart and Lung, 1971.

Chart XXXIII

CHOLESTEROL CONTENTS OF FOODS*

1. Meat, fish, and poultry
   mg/100 g (3.3 oz raw weight or 2.5 oz cooked weight)

Beef		Lamb		Pork	
Chuck Roast	55	Chops	66	Chops	55
Round Steak	68	Mutton	77	Ham	42
Rump Roast	58			Tenderloin	57
Tallow	56	Shellfish			
		Clams	49	Turkey	
Fish		Crab	99	dark meat	96
Codfish	46	Lobsters	83	light meat	61
Haddock	64	Oysters	59		
Halibut	33	Scallops	51	Chicken	
Herring	75	Shrimp	161	dark meat	76
Mackerel	80			light meat	54
Perch	63	Variety Meats			
Pike	71	Brains, Calf	1810	Veal	71
Salmon	55	Kidney	300		
Trout	57	Liver, Beef	320		
Tuna	51	Sweetbreads	280		

2. Cheeses
   mg/30 g (1 oz)

American	28	Cottage Cheese		Cream Cheese	42
American Process	26	Dry or Rinsed		Gouda (10% Fat)	10
Blue	47	1 ounce	1	Limburger	28
Cheddar	29	1/2 cup(90g)	1	Mozzarella	
Roquefort	22	Creamed		(part skim milk)	18
Swiss	27	1 ounce	5	Parmesan	
		1/2 cup(113g)	17	1 ounce	22
				1 tbls. (5g)	4

3. Dairy Products

Butter		Cream		Milk	
1 tsp. or pat(5g)	12	Thick or		mg/240g (1 cup)	
1/2 cup (120g)	299	whipping(heavy)		Buttermilk	14
		1 tbls. (15g)	21	Fortified Skim	
Egg		1/4 cup(60g)	84	(0.5% butterfat)	6
White	0	1/4 cup		Skim	2
1 Yolk	240	whipped(30g)	42	Whole	34
				2% butterfat	19

4. Fats

Lard		Margarine		Oils, Vegetable	0
1 tbls.	10	(vegetable)	0		
1/2 cup	78	Peanut butter	0		

*From Connor, Wm. E., Coronary Heart Disease Prevention Forum, Preventive Medicine, Vol. 1, No. 1, March 1972.

Chart XXXIV

CONTRAINDICATIONS TO EXERCISE AND EXERCISE TESTING

I. <u>Absolute Contraindications</u>

1. Manifest circulatory insufficiency ("Congestive Heart Failure")
2. Acute myocardial infarction
3. Active myocarditis
4. Rapidly increasing angina pectoris
5. Recent embolism, either systemic or pulmonary
6. Dissecting aneurysm
7. Acute infectious diseases
8. Thrombophlebitis
9. Ventricular tachycardia and other dangerous dysrhythmias (multifocal ventricular activity)
10. Severe aortic stenosis

II. <u>Relative Contraindications</u>[a]

1. Uncontrolled or high-rate supraventricular dysrhythmias
2. Repetitive or frequent ventricular ectopic activity
3. Untreated severe systematic or pulmonary hypertension
4. Ventricular aneurysm
5. Moderate aortic stenosis
6. Uncontrolled metabolic diseases (diabetes, thyrotoxicosis, Myxedema)
7. Severe myocardial obstructive syndromes (subaortic stenosis)
8. Marked cardiac enlargement
9. Toxemias of pregnancy

III. <u>Conditions requiring special consideration and/or precautions</u>

1. Conduction disturbances
   a. Complete atrioventricular block,
   b. Left bundle branch block,
   c. Wolff-Parkinson-White syndrome
2. Fixed rate pacemakers
3. Controlled dysrhythmias
4. Electrolyte disturbances
5. Certain medications
   a. Digitalis,
   b. B-blocking and drugs of related action
6. Clinically severe hypertension (Diastolic 110, Grade III retinopathy)
7. Angina pectoris and other manifestations of coronary insufficiency
8. Cyanotic heart disease
9. Intermittent or fixed right-to-left shunts
10. Severe anemia
11. Marked obesity
12. Renal, hepatic and other metabolic insufficiency
13. Overt psychoneurotic disturbances requiring therapy
14. Neuromuscular, musculoskeletal and arthritic disorders which would prevent activity

---

a In the practice of medicine the value of testing often exceeds the risk in patients with these relative contraindications. (From Samuel M. Fox, III, M.D., Preventive Medicine, Vol. 1, No. 1-2, March 1972, Acad. Press.)

Chart XXXV

ENERGY EXPENDITURES AT VARIOUS SPEEDS AND GRADES OF DIFFERENT TYPES OF PROGRESSION

Type of progression	Speed (m.p.h.)	Grade (%)	Energy expenditure 154-pound man	
			Calories per hour	Calories per mile
Horizontal walking	2.3	0	210	90
	3.5	0	290	85
	4.6	0	470	100
Grade walking	2.0	5.0	250	125
	2.5	5.0	290	115
	2.3	5.5	350	150
	3.5	5.5	450	130
	2.4	8.6	430	180
	3.5	8.6	560	160
Horizontal walking carrying 43 lb. load	1.0	0	210	210
	2.0	0	270	135
	3.0	0	350	115
	4.0	0	540	135
(Running)	5.0	0	820	165
Grade walking carrying 43 lb. load	0.5	35.8	370	740
	1.0	35.8	680	680
	1.5	35.8	890	595
Skiing along level	3.0	0	540	180
	5.0	0	720	145
	7.5	0	950	125
Swimming (breaststroke)	1.0		410	410
	1.6		490	305
	1.9		820	430

*Data is given as approximation from Morehouse & Miller, "Physiology of Exercise", C.V. Mosby, 1971.

Chart XXXVI

TRENDS IN AGE-ADJUSTED CANCER DEATH RATES
PER 100,000 POPULATION 1950-52 TO 1965-67

SEX	SITE	1950-52	1965-67	Percent Changes	COMMENTS
Male Female	All Sites All Sites	131.5 119.9	151.8 109.3	+15 - 9	Slight Increase Slight Decrease
Male Female	Breast Breast	0.2 21.8	0.2 22.8	- + 5	Constant Rate Slight Fluctuations: Overall No Change
Male Female	Colon & Rectum Colon & Rectum	19.2 18.3	18.9 16.1	- 2 -12	Slight Decrease in Both Sexes
Male Female	Lung Lung	19.7 4.0	40.6 6.8	+106 + 70	Steady Increase in Both Sexes Due to Cigarette Smoking
Male Female	Oral Oral	4.6 1.2	4.7 1.3	+ 2 + 8	Slight Fluctuation: Overall No Change Both Sexes
Male Female	Skin Skin	2.4 1.6	2.6 1.5	+ 8 - 6	Steady Slight Increase Slight Fluctuations: Overall No Change
Female	Uterus	21.8	11.5	- 47	Steady Decrease Attributed in Part to Widening Acceptance of Regular Checkup with "Pap Test."
Male Female	Esophagus Esophagus	3.8 0.9	4.1 1.0	+ 8 + 11	Slight Fluctuations: Overall No Change in Both Sexes
Male Female	Stomach Stomach	17.9 9.4	9.7 4.8	- 46 - 49	Steady Decrease in Both Sexes: Reasons Unknown
Male Female	Pancreas Pancreas	6.5 4.1	8.6 5.1	+ 32 + 24	Steady Increase in Both Sexes: Reasons Unknown
Male	Prostate	13.5	13.2	- 2	Early Increase, Later Decrease
Female	Ovary	6.8	7.6	+ 12	Steady Increase
Male Female	Kidney Kidney	2.8 1.6	3.4 1.6	+ 21 -	Steady Slight Increase Slight Fluctuation: Overall No Change
Male Female	Leukemia Leukemia	6.5 4.6	7.3 4.7	+ 12 + 2	Early Increase, Later Leveling Off Slight Early Increase, Later Leveling Off

*American Cancer Society - Cancer Journal for Clinicians Jan/Feb. 1971.

Chart XXXVII

<u>KNOW</u>

Cancer's Warning Signals!

<u>C</u> hange in bowel or bladder habits
<u>A</u> sore that does not heal
<u>U</u> nusual bleeding or discharge
<u>T</u> hickening or lump in breast or elsewhere
<u>I</u> ndigestion or difficulty in swallowing
<u>O</u> bvious change in wart or mole
<u>N</u> agging cough or hoarseness

If you have a warning signal, see your doctor.

BIBLIOGRAPHY

CHAPTERS I THROUGH VIII

Anstett, Patricia, "Maternal Nutrition Crusade Wins Support," Medical Tribune, Feb. 13, 1974.

Arena, Jay, "Children Must be Instructed Early About Hazards," Pediatric News, May 1972.

Aznor, R. and Bennett, A. E., "Pregnancy in the Adolescent," Am. J. Ob-Gyn, 81:934, 1961.

Babson, S. G. & Benson, Ralph, *Primer on Prematurity and High Risk Pregnancy*, C. V. Mosby Co. 1966.

Babson, S. G. and Phillips D. S. "Growth & Development of Twins Dissimilar in Size at Birth" New England Journal of Medicine, Vol. 289 #18, 937-40, November 1, 1973.

Babson, S. G. & Benson, Ralph, *Management of High Risk Pregnancy and Intensive Care of the Neonate*, C. V. Mosby Co., 1971.

Barker, Jane, "Infant Respiratory Crises May Cause Brain Damage," Medical Tribune, April 5, 1972.

Barnett, M. "Many of NYC's Abortions in Teen-Agers," Medical Tribune, February 6, 1974.

Bergner, L. and Susser, M. W., "Low Birth Weight and Prenatal Nutrition," Pediatrics, Vol. 46, No. 6.

Bond, C.B.Y., Dobbing, E. V., et al., *The Low Fat, Low Cholesterol Diet—What to Eat and How to Prepare It*, Doubleday & Co., Inc., 1971.

Brass, Irwin and Natarjan N., "Leukemia from Low Level Radiation: Identification of Susceptible Children," New England J. of Med., Vol. 287, July 20, 1972, Pg. 107-110.

Brewer, Tom, "Pregnancy and Nutrition, Part I, Current Opinion," Medical Tribune, July 26, 1972. "Part II," Medical Tribune, Aug. 2, 1972.

Brewer, Tom, "Society for Protection of the Unborn through Nutrition," 17 N. Wabash, Suite 604, Chicago, Illinois.

Caddell, J. L., "Magnesium Deprivation in Sudden Unexpected Infant Death," The Lancet, August 5, 1972.

Caffey, John, "The Parent-Infant Traumatic Stress Syndrome," Am. J. Roent. Rad, Therapy & Nuclear Med., Vol. 114, No. 2, Feb. 1972.

Callahan, Daniel, *The Great American Population Debate*, Doubleday, Inc. 1971. Contributing Authors listed as follows:

Bates, Marston, "Crowded People."
Blake, Judith, "Population Policy for America: Is Government Being Mislead."
Bogue, Donald, "The End of the Population Explosion."
Bumpass, Larry and Westoff, C., "Unwanted Births and U.S. Population Growth."
Chasteen, Edgar, "The Case for Compulsory Birth Control."
Coale, Ausley, "Man and His Environment."
Davis, Kingsley, "Population Policies: Will Current Programs Succeed."
Davis, Wayne, "Overpopulated Amreica."
Dyck, Arthur, "Population Policy and Ethical Acceptability."
Ehrlich, P. and Holdren, John, "Population & Environment."
Elliott, Robin, et al., "U.S. Population Growth and Family Planning A Revision of Literature."
Hardin, Garrett, "Multiple Paths to Population Control."
Harkavy, Oscar, et al., "Family Planning & Public Policy: Who is Misleading Whom?"
Ketchel, Melvin, "Fertility Control Agents as a Possible Solution to the World Population Problem."
Mayer, Jean, "Toward a Non-Malthusian Population Policy."
Norris, Kenneth, "The Third Fish."
Notestein, Frank, "Zero Population Growth. What is it?"
Poddock, Wm. and Paul, "Today Hungry Nations, Tomorrow Starving Nations."
Pollora, Frank, "Trends in U.S. Population."
Udall, Morris, "Spaceship Earth — Standing Room Only."
Wattenberg, Ben, "The Nonsense Explosion."

"Car Restraint Devices Designed for Children," American Academy of Pediatrics Newsletter, Report of Commission for Accident Prevention, February 1, 1972.

Charles, Seymour, "How Safe is Pupil Transportation?" Pediatrics, Vol. 45, No. 1, Part II, Jan. 1970.

"Chart Book on Smoking," U.S. Dept. of Health, Education and Welfare, Printing Office, 1969.

Cherry, B. J., et al., "Obstacles to Delivery of Medical Care to Children of Neglecting Parents," Am. J. Public Health, 61:567-73, March, 1971.

"Childhood Diet and Coronary Heart Disease," Pediatrics, Vol. 49, No. 2, February, 1972.

Coggle, J. E., *Biological Effects of Radiation*, Wykeham Pub. (London) Ltd. 1971, Springer-Verlag, N.Y. Inc.

"Continued Decline in Infant Mortality," American Medical News, Aug. 20, Sept. 10 and Nov. 5, 1973.

Cooper, Kenneth H., *A New Aerobic*, Bantam Books, 1970.

Cooper, Mildred, *Aerobics for Women*, M. Evans & Co., 1972.

Cooper, Louis, "Rubella — A Preventable Cause of Birth Defects," Birth Defects, National Foundation of March of Dimes, Dec. 1968.

Coyne, Martin, "The Battered Child Syndrome," Parts I, II, III, & IV, Minn. Med., 51:1793-9, Dec. 1968, 52:155-6 345-7; 539-40, Jan., Feb. & March, 1969.

Curran, W. J. and Hyg, S. M., "An Enigma Wrapped in Swaddling Clothes; Congress and Crib Death," New Eng. J. Med. 287:235-37, Aug. 3, 1972.

Dahl, L. K. and Love, R. A., "Etiological Role of Sodium Chloride Intake in Essential Hypertension in Humans," J.A.M.A. 164:397-400, 1957.

Done, Helen K., et al., "Evaluation of Safety Packaging for Protection of Children," Pediatrics, Vol. 48, Oct. 1971.

Drash, Allen, "Arteriosclerosis, Cholesterol, and the Pediatrician," J. of Ped., Vol. 80, April, 1972.

Drillien, C. M., "Etiology and Prognosis of Small for Date Infant," Pediatric Clinics of North America, Vol. 17, No. 1.

Ehrlich, Paul R., *The Population Bomb*, Ballantine Books, 1968.

Ehrlich, Paul R. and Ehrlich, Anna H., *Population Resources Environment Issues in Human Ecology*, W. H. Freeman, Inc., 1970.

"Fatal Accidents Among School Age Children," Statistical Bulletin, Metropolitan Life Insurance Company, Vol. 54, Dec. 1973.

Faulkner, Frank, "Placental Influence on Fetal Development," Pediatric Clinics of North America, Vol. 17, No. 1, Small for the Date Infant.

Fleck, Stephen, "Child Abuse and Abortion," Editorial, Med. Tribune, Aug. 2, 1972.

Fleet, W. F., Jr., et al., "Fetal Consequences of Maternal Rubella Immunizations," J.A.M.A. Feb. 11, 1974, Vol. 227 No. 6, 621-27.

Fort, A. T., et al., "Counseling the Patient with Sickle Cell Disease About Reproduction – Pregnancy and Its Outcome Does Not Justify the Maternal Risk," Am. J. Obst. & Gyn. 111:324-7, Oct. 1971.

Franciosi, R. A., et al., "Some Newborns' Congenital Infections can be Prevented by Treating Mother," Med. Tribune, April 5, 1972.

Friedman, Glenn, "Detection of Risk of Atherosclerosis in Children Urged," Med. Tribune, March 15, 1972.

Friedman, Glenn, "Low Fat Diet Safe For Youngsters," Med. Tribune, Dec. 19, 1973.

Gibson, R., et al., "Leukemia in Children Exposed to Multiple Risk Factors," New Eng. J. Med., Vol. 279, No. 17, pp. 906-9.

Gil, David, "Physical Abuse of Children," Nationwide Survey, Pediatrics 44: Suppl. 857-64, Nov. 1969.

Gilfillan, R. F., "Current Status of Rubella Susceptibility Testing," New Eng. J. Med., 286:320-21, Feb. 10, 1972.

Glass, Leonard, et al., "Effect of Heroin Withdrawal on Respiratory Rate and Acid-Base Status in the Newborn," New Eng. J. of Med., April 6, Vol. 286, No. 14.

Glueck, C. J., et al., "Hyperlipemia in Progeny of Parents with Myocardial Infarction Before Age 50," Am. J. Dis. of Children, Vol. 127 No. 1, 70-8, 1974.

Gordon, H. H., "The Infants of Diabetic Mothers," Am. J. of Med. Science, 244:129-144, July, 1962.

Gordon, H. H., Albert Einstein College of Medicine, Lecture at Daniel C. Darrow Lectureship, March 7, 1972, Kansas City, Mo.

Gresham, Edwin L., "Special Center will Treat High Risk Infants," AMA News, January 17, 1972.

Gubner, Richard, "Stop Ma – You're Killing Me," Med. Tribune, June 28, 1972.

Hall, Wesley W., "Health is Everybody's Business," Am. Med. News, April 17, 1972.

Hammouda, A. A., "Caesarean Section in the Young Gravida – A 10 Year Analysis," Am. J. Ob. & Gyn., 100:267-9, Jan. 1968.

Hanshaw, James, "Congenital Cytomegalovirus Infection," Birth Defects, National Foundation March of Dimes, Dec. 1968.

Hardy, Janet, "Import of Low Birth Weight Key Perinatal Study Finding," Med. Tribune, Vol. 13, No. 2, Jan. 12, 1972.

Haworth, James C., "Smoke Effect on Size of Fetal Body and Brain," Med. Tribune, March 29, 1972.

Hirsch, Jules, "Can We Modify the Number of Adipose Cells," Post Grad. Med., 51:83-86.

Holsten, Donald H., "Organic Food A Fraud?" New Eng. J. of Med., Aug. 12, 1971.

"Infant Mortality Rate Continued Decline 1971," AMA News, 2/21/72.

"Impact of the Tumbling Birth Rate: Three Views," AMA News, July 17, 1972.

Jablon, S. and Kato, H., "Childhood Cancer in Relation to Prenatal Exposure to Atomic Bomb Radiation," Lancet, Vol. II, 1000-03.

James, George, "Preventive Medicine: Management of the Disease Process," Preventive Med., Vol. 1:15-19, March 1972.

Janiciki, Ed, "What You Should Know About Safety Seats," Midwest Motorist, June 1972.

Johnson, R. T., "Effects of Viral Infection on the Developing Nervous System," New Eng. J. Med., 287:599-604, Sept., 12, 1971.

Jokl, Ernest, *Physiology of Exercise*, Charles Thomas Pub. 1964.

Kane, Sydney, "Advancing Age and the Premigravida," Ob. & Gyn. 29: 409-414, March 1967.

Kannel, W. V. and Dawer, Thomas, "Atherosclerosis as a Pediatric Problem," J. of Ped., Vol. 80, April 1972.

Katz, Samuel, and Kurgman, Saul, "Pediatricians Back Proposals to Drop Small Pox Vaccination," Med. Tribune, Dec. 15, 1971.

Keys, A., et al., "Coronary Heart Disease in Seven Countries," Circulation Supplement, Vol. 41-42, 1970.

Kirschbaum, Thomas H., et al., "Some Acute Effects of Smoking in Sheep and Their Fetus," Ob. & Gyn., Vol. 35, 1970.

Kirschbaum, Thomas H., et al., "Diseases You Can Get From Your Pets," Ob. & Gyn., Vol. 35, 1970.

Kuller, Lewis, "Sudden Death in Arteriosclerotic Heart Disease; A Case For Preventive Medicine," Am. J. Cardiology, Nov. 1969.

Lele, P. P., "No Chromosomal Damage from Ultrasound," New Eng. J. of Med., 287:254, Aug. 3, 1972.

Lubchenco, L. O., et al., "Long Term Follow-up of Prematurely Born Infants," J. of Ped., Vol. 80, No. 3.

MacMahan, Brian, "Etiology of Congenital Defects," New Eng. J. of Med., 287-514, September 7, 1972.

Maragos, George, et al., "Accidental Poisoning of Children in Transit," J. of Ped., July, 1971.

Marak, E. M., "Agricultural Chemicals as Pollutants," *Proc. Western Hemisphere Nutrition Congress III*, Futura Publ. Co. 1971.

Miller, Herbert C., "Diagnosis of Impaired Fetal Growth in New Born Infants," Pediatrics, Vol. 48, No. 4, Oct. 1971.

Mitchell, Sheila and Cooper, Theodore, "Preventive Medicine: The Approximation of Paradise?" Prev. Med., Vol. 1:15-19, Mar. 1972.

Monthly Vital Statistics of United States, Vol. 20 No. 13, August 30, 1972.

Moriyama, Iwo, et al., *Cardiovascular Diseases in United States*, Harvard University Press, 1971.

Nadler, Henry, "Combating Neonatal Mortality," Pediatric News, May, 1972.

National Tuberculosis and Respiratory Disease Association, "The First Breath," Dec. 1969, Vol. 42, No. 10.

Naeye, Richard, "Malnutrition, Probable Causes of Fetal Growth Retardation," Archives of Pathology, Vol. 79, March 1965.

Naeye, Richard L., and Blanc, W. A., "Autopsy Records of 1004 Neonates Show Ill Effects of High Risk Mothers," Med. Tribune, Vol. 13, No. 15, August 12, 1972.

Paffenbarger, R. S., "Characteristics of Youth Predisposing to the Fatal Stroke in Later Years," Lancet, April 8, 1967.

Pasner, N. A., et al., "Outcome of Pregnancy in Class A Diabetics," Am. J. Obst-Gyn. IV 886-95, Dec. 1971.

Pasternack, S. A., "Hand Guns and Homicide," Med. Tribune, Jan. 23, 1974.

Paull, Dorothy, et al., "A New Approach to Reporting Child Abuse," Hospitals, Jol. Am. Hosp. Assn., 41:62-64.

Pildes, R. S., "Infants of Diabetic Mothers," New Eng. Jol. Med. Vol. 289, No. 17, 902-4, October 25, 1973.

Pleas, et al., "Prevention of Injuries to Children in Automobiles," Pediatrics, Vol. 49, No. 3, Mar. 1972.

"Problems Created by Medical Progress," Medical World News, April 7, 1972.

"Reducing Infant Mortality Rates," National Center for Health Statistics, Feb. 28, 1972.

Remington, Jack, "Toxoplasmosis and Congenital Infection," Birth Defects, National Foundation March of Dimes, Dec. 1968.

Reynolds, D. W., et al., "Maternal Cytomegalovirus Excretion and Perinatal Infection," New Eng. Jol. Med., Vol. 289 No. 1, July 5, 1973, 1-4.

Robinson, D. "Sickle Cell – Point, Counterpoint," New Eng. Jol. Med. Vol. 289, No. 6, 323-24, August 6, 1973.

Roth, Russell B., "Emphasis on Preventive Medicine Disputed by Dr. Roth," AMA News, March 27, 1972.

Sackler, A.M., "Doomsday, The Population Bomb and the Pill," Med. Tribune, Feb. 6, 1974.

Sanderson, Eric, "Frank Facts for Fat Folks," Modern Medicine, Nov. 1969.

Scherz, R. G., "Prevention of Childhood Aspirin Poisoning," New Eng. J. of Med. 285:1361-62, Dec. 9, 1971.

Scott, Robert, "Profile of Sickle Cell Disease," JAMA. Vol. 214 No. 4, Oct. 1970.

Seelig, R. A., "Organically Grown Foodstuffs," JAMA, Vol. 220, No. 6, 5-8-72, pp. 866.

Shank, R. E., "The Ecology of Malnutrition – Examples of Host Factors," *Proc. West Hemisphere Nutrition Congress III.*

Shepard, F. M., et al., "Residual Pulmonary Findings in Clinical Hyaline-Membrane Disease," New Eng. J. Med. 279:1063-70, Nov. 14, 1968.

Silver, Larry, et al., "Child Abuse Syndrome – Gray Areas in Diagnosis," Ped. Vol. 44, No. 4, Oct. 1969.

Silver, Larry, et al., "Child Battery: Seek and Save," Medical World News, 6-2-72.

Singer, Dale, "Crib Death," St. Louis Univ. Magazine, Vol. 45, No. 4.

Smith, C. A., "The Battered Child," New England Jol. Med. Vol. 229, No. 6, Aug. 9, 1973, 322-23.

"Sterilization Guidelines: 22 Months on the Shelf," Med. World News. Nov. 9, 1973.

Stewart, Alice, and Kneale, G. W., "Radiation Dose Effects Relation to Obstetrics, X-rays and Childhood Cancers," Lancet, Vol. 1, June 6, 1970.

"Survey Reveals Midwesterners Healthiest," Greater Kansas City Medical Bulletin, June 1, 1972.

Swift, PGF & Emery, J., "Magnesium and Sudden Unexpected Infant Death," Lancet, No. 7782, Vol. II, 1972, Page 871.

Thatcher, Robert A., "Genetic Counseling for Sickle Cell Disease Carriers," New Eng. J. of Med., Nov. 25, 1971.

The High Cost of Childhood, Esquire, March, 1974.

Underwood, et al., "Effect of Smoking on Fetal Development," Obst. & Gyn., Vol. 29, 1967, Page 1.

Vital Statistics of the United States, General Mortality, Vol. II, 1967.

Vital Statistics of the United States, Natality, Vol. 1, 1967, Superintendent of Documents.

Valdes-Dapena, Maria, et al., "Myocardial Conduction System in Sudden Death in Infancy," New Eng. Jol. Med. Vol. 289, 1179, Nov. 29, 1973.

Wagner, Susan, *Cigarette Country*, Prager, 1971.

Waller, Julian, "Bicycle Ownership Use and Injury Patterns Among Elementary School Chidlren," Pediatrics, Vol. 47, No. 6, June 1971.

Weller, T. H., "The Cytomegaloviruses, 2 Parts," New Eng. J. of Med. 285: 203-14, July 22, 1971.

Winick, Myron, "Cellular Growth and Intra-uterian Malnutrition," Pediatric Clinics of North America, Vol. 17, No. 1, Small for the Date Infant.

Wise, George, "Poison Prevention," Children's Mercy Hospital Lecture, Kansas City, Missouri, 1972.

Wollman, D. H. M., "Effects of Environment Factors on the Fetus," Birth Defects Reprint Series, National Foundation of the March of Dimes.

Zelson, Carl, et al., "Neonatal Narcotic Addiction," Pediatrics, Vol. 48, No. 2, Aug. 1971.

Zeron, Z. M., "Etiology of Crib Death," New Eng. Jol. Med. Vol. 289, 1252-3, Dec. 1973.

CHAPTER IX

Beedleman, Barkley, "Hazards of Marijuana," New Eng. J. of Med., 386: 1157-8, May 25, 1972.

Briggs, T.G., "Alcoholism as a Disease," AMA News, July 3, 1972.

Campbell, Horace, "Automotive Safety," Medical Tribune, Apr. 1972, July 1972.

Constostovlos, D.L., "Renewed Interest in Gun Control," New Eng. J. of Med. 285:1091-92, Nov. 4, 1971.

Cracchiolo III, Andrea, et al, "Motorcycle Injuries to University Students," JAMA, Vol. 204, No. 1, pg. 175-77, April 1, 1968.

Craig, T.T., *Comments in Sports Medicine*, AMA Educ, Press 1973.

Douglass, John, "Protection of Automobile Occupants," American Family Physician, Vol. 4, No. 6, pg. 117-24, 1971.

Glaser, Kurt, "Suicidal Children – Management," Am. J. of Psycho. Therapy, Vol. 25, No. 1, Pg. 27-36, Jan. 1971.

Hanson, Jerome, Simons, John, "Alcohol-Related Highway Accidents," Minn. Med., Vol. 53, No. 8, pg. 905-7.

Kolansky, Harold & Moore, W.T., "Toxic Effects of Chronic Marijuana Use," JAMA, Vol. 222:35-41.

McDermott, John, "The Car Clinic," Medical Tribune, May 10, 1972.

McIntire, Matilda and Angle, Carol, "The Toxonomy of Suicide as Seen in Poison Control Centers," Ped. Clinics of North Am., Vol. 17, No. 3, Pg. 697, Aug. 1970.

Malmquist, C.P., "Depressions in Childhood and Adolescence – Two Parts," New Eng. J. Med., 284:887-93, April 22, 1971, April 29, 1971.

"Medical Aspects of Motorcycle Safety," Committee on Medical Aspects of Automotive Safety, JAMA, Vol. 205, No. 5, pg. 92-3, July 29, 1968.

Metropolitan Life Statistical Bulletin

(a) "Hazardous Avocations," June 1970.

(b) "Mortality from Accidents in Canada and the United States," June 1973.

(c) "Mortality from Home Accidents," Vol. 54, March 1973.

(d) "Motorcycle Accident Fatalities," Vol. 54, Aug. 1973.

(e) "Regional Variations in Mortality from Suicide," Vol. 54, Aug. 1973.

Morrison, Robert, "Agnew, Alcohol, Automobiles & Assessment," Science, Vol. 169, #3948, Aug. 1970.
Naham, Allen, et al, "Types of Fatal Accidents," International Conf. on Accident Pathology, Washington 1968.
Nelson, Gaylord, "Tires and Automotive Safety," Medical Tribune, March 1, 1972.
Nicholi, Armand M., "The Motorcycle Syndrome," Am. J. Psychiat., Vol. 126:11, pg. 1588-95, May 1970.
Pyle, Howard, "Safety Belts – Real Preventive Medicine in Automotive Safety," Prev. Med., Vol. 2, No. 1, March 1973.
"Researchers 'Rev Up' for Safer Driving," Editorial, JAMA, Vol. 219, No. 8, Feb. 21, 1972.
Robinson, Derek, "Pass at Your Own Risk," New Eng. J. Med., 286: 1157-8, May 25, 1972.
Ross, Mathew, "Suicide Among College Students," Am. J. of Psychiat., Vol. 126, No. 2, Pg. 220-25, Aug. 1969.
Schechter, Marshall & Sternlof, Richard, "Suicide in Adolescents," Post Grad. Med., Vol. 49, pg. 220-23, 1970.
Shapiro, H.A., "Alcohol and Traffic Safety," J. of Forensic Med. Vol. 17, No. 4, pg. 133-35.
Shapiro, H.A., "Alcohol and the Halocaust on Our Roads," J. Forensic Med., Vol. 17, No. 1, pg. 1-4.
"Stresses of Life Making Young Men and Women High Risks for Suicide," Medical Tribune, Vol. 13, No. 15, Apr. 12, 1972.
Sturner, W.Q., "Drinking, Driving and Dying," New Eng. J. of Med., 284:160-161, Jan. 21, 1971.
"Suicide – A Tragic Toll but Still a Taboo Topic," Am. Med. News, Dec. 17, 1973. .
U.S. News & World Report, "News You Can Use," Jan. 24, 1972.
Vital Statistics of the United States, *General Mortality*, Vol. II, Superintendant of Documents, U.S. Govt. Printing Office, 1967.
Walker, Earl, "Head Injuries" (Personal Communication Dr. Charles Brackett, Kansas University Professor of Neurosurgery).
Waller, Julian, "Medical Conditions – What Role in Crashes?," New Eng. J. of Med., pg. 429-30, Aug. 20, 1970.

CHAPTER X

Alcoholic Cirrhosis and Other Toxic Hepatopathies, S. Randia International, Ed. Engle, Arthur & Larsson, Tage, Nordiska Bokhendelns Forlag, 1970.
(a) Bonnichsen, R., "Liver Alcohol Dehydrogenase"
(b) Forsander, O.A., "The Effect of Ethanol on Liver Metabolism"
(c) Hallin, J. and Linne, I., "Cirrhosis of Liver in One Community"
(d) Leevy, C.M., "Hard Liquor and Cirrhosis"
(e) Martini, G.A., Bode, C.H., "Epidemiology of Cirrhosis of Liver"
(f) Moeschlin, S. and Righetti, P., "Wine and Cirrhosis"

Beaconsfield, Peter, et al., "Marijuana Smoking: Cardiovascular Effects in Man and Possible Mechanisms," New Eng. J. Med. 287:209-212, Aug. 3, 1972.

Chafetz, Morris (Chairman of Task Force), "Alcohol and Health" – First Report to the U.S. Congress from Sec. HEW, HEW Pub., Dec. 1971. (#72-9099, Supt. of Documents, U.S. Printing Office Stocks #1724-0193).

Chafetz, Morris, "Alcoholism Prevention and Reality," Quart. J. Stud. Alc., 28:345-349, 1967.

Davidson, Charles, *Liver Pathophysiology: Its Revelance to Human Disease*, Little, Brown & Co. 1970.

DeLint, Jan, "The Prevention of Alcoholism," Prev. Med., Vol. 3, No. 1, pg. 24-35, March 1974.

Gould, Lawrence, et al., "Cardiac Effects of a Cocktail," JAMA 218:1799-1802, Dec. 20, 1971.

Laurie, W., "Alcoholism Held Responsible for 3% of Australian Deaths," Med. Tribune, March 8, 1972.

Major, R., *A History of Medicine*, Vol. II, Charles Thomas Pub.

"Narcotics and Alcoholism," Hearings before Subcommittee on Labor and Public Welfare, U.S. Senate, Part I, U.S. Govt. Printing Office.

Popham, Robert (Editor), *Alcohol and Alcoholism*, International Symposium in Memory of E.M. Jellinek, Univ. of Toronto Press 1970.

Read, A.E. (Editor), *The Liver Symposium of the Colston Research Society*, Univ of Bristol, Pub. Butterworths – London, 1967.

Senior, John, "Ethenol and Liver Disease," Post Grad. Med. Series, Diseases of Liver, McGraw Hill 1968.

Tashero, M. and Lipscomb, W.F., "Mortality experiences of Alcoholics," Quart. J. Stud. Alc. 24:203-212, 1963.

Vital Statistics of the United States, *General Mortality*, Vol. II, Superintendant of Documents, 1967.

CHAPTER XI

Anderson, E.W., "Low CO Levels Worsen Heart Ischemia," Med. Tribune, July 19, 1972.

Astrand, Per-Olaf & Rodale, K., *Textbook of Work Physiology*, McGraw-Hill, 1970.

Bassler, T., Newsletter, American Medical Joggers Assn., March 1973.

Beard, Earl, "11% of Exercised Executives Develop Cardiac Arrhythmias," Medical Tribune, June 7, 1972.

Berne, Robert and Levy, Matthew, *Cardiovascular Physiology*, C.V. Mosby & Co., 1972.

Berry, Maxwell, "Pathogenesis of Atherosclerosis," *The Third Trimester*, Pub. Maxwell Berry, 1971.

Best, Charles H. and Taylor, Norman B., *Physiological Basis of Medical Practice*, Williams & Wilkins Publishers.

Blackburn, H., "Prognostic Importance of Premature Beats Following Myocardial Infarct," JAMA 223:116, Mar. 5, 1973.

Borgotta, Edgar & Evans, Robert, *Smoking Health & Behavior,* Aldine Pub. Co., Chicago.

Boyer, J.L., "Prevention and Rehabilitation in Coronary Heart Disease," The Physician and Sports Medicine, Vol. 2, No. 1, pg. 41-45, Jan. 1974.

Chatterjee, Kance, et al., "Depression of Left Ventricular Function Due to Myocardial Ischemia and Its Reversal After Aortocoronary Saphenous Vein By-pass," New Eng. J. of Med. 286-1117-1122, May 25, 1972.

Christakis, George and Rathmann, Dorothy, "Position Statement of American Health Foundation on Diet and Coronary Heart Disease," Prev. Med., Vol. 1:255-286, March 1972.

Connor, William E., and Connor, Sonja, "The Key Role of Nutritional Factors in the Prevention of Coronary Heart Disease," Prev. Med. Vol. 1:49-83, March 1972.

Cooper, K.H., "Testing and Developing Cardiovascular Fitness," J. Phy. Education, Mar.-Apr. 1972.

Cooper, K.H., *New Aerobics*, Evans & Lippencott, New York, 1970.

Cooper, K.H., *Aerobics*, J. B. Lippencott, New York, 1968.

Cooper, Theodore, "10 Year Study of Factors in Heart Disease is Urged," Med. Tribune, Jan. 26, 1972.

Cranefield, P.F., "Ventricular Fibrillation," New Eng. J. Med., Vol. 289 No. 14, pg. 732-36, Oct. 4, 1973.

Cureton, T.K., *The Physiological Effects of Exercise Programs on Adults,* C.C. Thomas Pub. 1969.

Cureton, T.K., "Physical Fitness and Dynamic Health," Jol. of Phys. Educ. Mar.-Apr. 1972.

Daniell, Harry, "Osteoporosis and Smoking," JAMA, 221:509, July 31, 1972.

"Diet and Heart Disease," American Heart Association, 10-68-200m 1968.

"Evaluation for Exercise Participation," AMA Committee on Exercise and Physical Fitness, JAMA 219:900-01, Feb. 14, 1972.

Falls, H.B., *Exercise Physiology*, Academic Press, New York, 1968.

Fletcher, Charles, "New Scientific Data on Smoking," Nat. Conf. on Smoking, Health, San Diego, Calif. Sept. 1970.

Fox, Samuel III, "Physical Activity and the Prevention of Coronary Heart Disease," Bulletin of New York Acad. Med. 44:950, 1966.

Fox, S.M. III & Naughton, J.P., "Physical Activity and Prevention of Coronary Heart Disease," Prev. Med., Vol. 1, 92-120, 1972.

Fox, S.M. III and Haskell, W.L., "Physical Activity and Health Maintenance," Journal of Rehab. 32:89-92, 1966.

Fox, Samuel III, et al, "Physical Activity and the Prevention of Coronary Heart Disease," Annals of Clinical Research, 3:404-432, 1971.

Fox, Samuel III, "Life to Your Years – And Possibly Years to Your Life," Jol. Phy. Education, Mar. & Apr. 1972.

Fulton, Julian O., "Research on Acute Myocardial Infarction," Suppl. IV to Circ., Vol. 39 & 40, Nov. 1969.

Golding, L.A., "Cholesterol and Exercise," Jol. of Phy. Educ., Mar. & Apr. 1972.

Goldman, Arthur et al, "Body Habitus and Serum Cholesterol in Essential Hypertension and Renovascular Hypertension," JAMA, Vol. 221, No. 4, pg. 378-83, July 24, 1972.

Goldstein, Samuel, "The Biology of Aging," New Eng. J. of Med., 285: 1120-29, Nov. 11, 1971.

Harvey, Norman, "In Praise of Exercise," New Eng. J. of Med. 286:323, Feb. 10, 1972.

Helfant, R.H. et al, "Functional Importance of the Human Coronary Collateral Circulation," New Eng. J. of Med., 284:1277-31, June 10, 1971.

Hellerstein, H.K. & Friedman, E.H., "Sexual Activity and the Post-Coronary Patient," Med. Aspects Human Sexuality, 3:70, 1969.

Jick, H., et al, "Coffee and Myocardial Infarction," New Eng. J. of Med., Vol. 289, pg. 63-67, July 12, 1973.

Jick, H., et al, "Coffee Drinking and Myocardial Infarction," JAMA, Vol. 227, pg. 801-803, (Includes rebuttal by Klatsky, et al), Feb. 18, 1974.

Jokl, Ernst, "Exercise and Cardiac Death," JAMA 218:1707, 1971.

Jokl, Ernst, *Physiology of Exercise*, Charles Thomas Pub. 1964.

Kannel, W.B. et al, "Physical Activity and Coronary Vulnerability: The Framingham Study," Cardiology Digest, Vol. 6, pg. 28-40, 1971.

Kannel, William, "Lipid Profile and the Potential Coronary Victim," Am. J. Cl. Nutrition, 24:1074-81, Sept. 1971.

Kannel, William and McNamare, P.R., "The Evidence for Excess Risk," Minn. Med., Vol. 52:1197-1201, Aug. 1969.

Kannel, William, "Coffee and Coronary Disease," New Eng. Jol. Med., Vol. 289, pg. 100-01, July 12, 1973.

Klatsky, A.L., et al, "Coffee Drinking Prior to Acute Myocardial Infarction," JAMA, Vol. 226, No. 5, pg. 540-43, Oct. 29, 1973.

Langer, G.A., "The Intrinsic Control of Myocardial Contraction—Ionic Factors," New Eng. J. of Med., Vol. 285, No. 19, pg. 1065-71.

Levy, Robert, "Hyperlipoproteinema," JAMA, Vol. 226, No. 6, pg. 648-49, Nov. 5, 1973.

"Link Between Stress, Infarct Said to Have Been Identified," Hospital Tribune, Sept. 4, 1972.

Major, Ralph, *A History of Medicine*, Vol. II Charles Thomas & Co.

Miettinen, M. et al, "Effect of Cholesterol-lowering Diet on Mortality from Coronary Heart Disease and Other Causes," Lancet, #7782, Vol. II, pg. 835-38, 1972.

Morehouse, L.E. & Miller, A.T., *Physiology of Exercise*, 6th Edition, C.V. Mosby Co., St. Louis, 1971.

Morris, J.N., et al, "Vigorous Exercise in Leisure Time and Incidence of Coronary Heart Disease," Lancet, Feb. 1972.

Morse, R.L., *Exercise and the Heart*, Charles Thomas Pub., 1972.

Page, I.H. and Stamler, J., "Diet and Coronary Heart Disease," Parts I & II, Modern Concepts of Cardiovascular Disease 27:119-123; 125-128, Sept.-Oct. 1968.

Page, I.H., "Get Off Your Fatty Acids," Modern Medicine, May 19, 1969.

Pepine, C.J., "Severe Coronary Disease Seen in Asymptomatic Young Men," Med. Tribune, July 12, 1972.

Raab, Wilhelm, *Preventive Myocardiology*, Charles C. Thomas, 1970.

Redwood, D.R., "Circulatory and Symptomatic Effects of Physical Training in Patients with Coronary Artery Diseases and Angina Pectoris," New Eng. J. of Med. 286:959-64.

Reeves, T.J. and Sheffield, L.T., "The Influence of Age and Athletic Training on Maximal Heart Rate During Exercise," from *Coronary Heart Disease and Physical Fitness*, Univ. Park Press, Baltimore, Md.

Reeves, T.J., et al, "Exercise Tests," JAMA 221-1165, Sept. 4, 1972.

Reid, D.D., "Smoking and Ischemic Heart Disease Prevention – Problems and Potential," Prev. Med., Vol. 1:84-91, Mar. 1972.

Simonson, Ernest, *Physiology of Work Capacity and Fatigue*, Chas. Thomas Pub. 1971.

"Smoking and Health," Summary and Report of the Royal College of Physicians of London on Smoking in Relation to Cancer of Lung and Other Diseases, Pitman Pub. Co., New York.

Sneddon, Russell C., "Physical Fitness for Exercise Participation," JAMA, Vol. 220, No. 4, pg. 589, April 24, 1972.

Spain, D.M., et al, "Women Smokers and Sudden Death," JAMA, Vol. 224, pg. 1005-07, May 14, 1973.

Stamler, Jeremiah, "Primary Prevention of Acute Myocardial Infarction," Mod. Medicine, Oct. 5, 1970.

Stamler, J. and Epstein, F.H., "Coronary Heart Disease: Risk Factors as Guide to Preventive Action," Preventive Medicine, Vol. 1:27-48, March 1972.

"Survival Among Insured Men Following Disability From Coronary Heart Disease," Metropolitan Life Statistical Bulletin, June 1970.

"The Big Three Risk Factors that Predict Coronary Disease Best," Med. World News, Nov. 9, 1973.

Vital Statistics of the United States, *General Mortality*, Vol. II, Superintendant of Documents, 1967.

Wissler, R.W., "Definitive Study Ties U.S. Diet, Atherosclerosis," Med. Tribune, Dec. 15, 1971.

Wynder, Ernest & Hill, Peter, "Blood Lipids: How Normal is Normal," Preventive Med., Vol. 1:161-166.

Wynder, E.L., "Etiological and Preventive Aspects of Human Cancer," Prev. Med., Vol. 1, No. 3, pg. 300-334, 1972.

Zakel, W.J., "A Short Term Community Study of the Epidemiology of Coronary Heart Disease," Am. J. Pub. Health 49:1630-39.

Zohman, Lenora R., "Marital Sex Believed to be Safe in Patients with Heart Disease," Med. Tribune, Mar. 29, 1972.

CHAPTER XII

Ashley, David and Davies, H.D., "Lung Cancer in Women," Thorax, Vol. 24, No. 4, July 1969.

Auerbach, Oscar, et al, "Relationship of Smoking and Age to Emphysema: Whole Lung Section Study," New Eng. J. of Med. 286:853-57, Apr. 20, 1972.

Bates, D.V., et al, *Respiratory Function in Disease*, 2nd Edition, W.B. Saunders Co. 1971.

Berry, Maxwell, "Cigarette Smoking," *The Third Trimester*, Publ. Maxwell Berry, 1971.

Boucot, K.R., et al, "Screening for Lung Cancer," JAMA, Vol. 226, No. 5, pg. 556-57, Oct. 29, 1973.

Carnow, Bertram, et al, "The Role of Air Pollution in Chronic Obstructive Pulmonary Disease," JAMA 214:894-99, Nov. 2, 1970.

"Cigarette Consumption Statistics," Am. Med. News, Nov. 19, 1973.

Cotes, J.E., *Lung Function*, 2nd Edition, F.A. Davis Co., Philadelphia.

Finch, C.A. and Lenfant, C., "Oxygen Transport in Man," New Eng. J. of Med. 286:407-415.

Gregg, Ian, "Bronchitis: Familiarity Has Bred Contempt," Med. Tribune, Jan. 26, 1972.

Hoffmann, D., "Tobacco Smoke Compared to Air Polution," Preventive Med., Vol. 1, No. 3, pg. 450, Aug. 1972.

Kazemi, Homayoun, "Pulmonary Function Tests," JAMA 206:2302-04.

Larson, Roger et al, "Genetic and Environmental Determinants of Chronic Obstructive Lung Disease," Abstracts – Nat. Foundation T.B. and Resp. Diseases, Vol. 43, No. 8.

Levine, Harold, "Physiology of Cigarette Smoke," Lecture St. Luke's Hospital, Kansas City, Mo., 1972 and Personal Communication.

Prute, Philip, "Autopsy Study of Emphysema Supports Antismoking Advice," Med. Tribune, Jan 26, 1972.

Rubin, Philip, "Moments of Decision in Lung Cancer," Pub. Am. Coll. Radiology, 1971.

Steinfeld, J.L., (U.S. Surgeon General), "Report by Public Health Service Cites Effects of Smoking on Non-smoker," Med. Tribune, Feb. 2, 1972.

Tashkin, O.P. et al, "Acute Pulmonary Physiology Effects of Smoked Marijuana and Oral D9-Tetrahydrocannabinol in Healthy Young Men," New England J. of Med., Vol. 289, No. 7, pg. 336-41, Aug. 7, 1973.

Terry, Luther, "Smoking and Health," Report of Advisory Committee to the Surgeon General of Public Health Service, U.S. Govt. Printing Office, #1103, 1964.

Weiss, William, "X-Ray Screening No Prognosis Aid in Lung Cancers," Med. Tribune, July 26, 1972.

U.S. Dept. Health, Education and Welfare, "Bibliography on Smoking and Health," Part I and II, 1969. (7000 references), Pub. Health Service Pub. #1124, May 1969 and June 1970.

Vital Statistics of the United States, *General Mortality*, Vol. II, Superintendant of Documents, 1967.

CHAPTER XIII

Ahluwalia, H.S., and Doll, R., Brit. Jol. Prev. Soc. Med. 22, pg. 161, 1968.

Allen, D.W., and Cole, P., "Viruses and Human Cancer," New England J. of Med., Vol. 286, No. 2, pg. 70-86.

Breslow, Lester, "Early Case Finding, Treatment and Mortality From Cervix and Breast Cancer," Prev. Med., Vol. 1, No. 1 & 2, pg. 141-52.

Ca – A Cancer Journal for Clinicians, Am. Cancer Soc., Jan./Feb. 1974.

1974 Cancer Facts and Figures, Am. Cancer Soc.

"Cancer Study Finds Changes in U.S. Rates in 22 Year Period," Med. Tribune, Jan. 26, 1972.

Carter, Barham, *Cerebral Infarction,* The Macmillan Co. 1964.

Chamberlin, Richard H., et al, "The Carcinogenic Hazard of Radiation to the Breasts," Ca – Can. Jol. for Clinicians, 20:24-31, Jan.-Feb. 1970.

Clark, R.L., Cumley, R.W., et al, "Oncology 1970," Vol. II, *Treatment and Management of Cancer*, YearBook Publishers 1971.

Coggle, J.E., *Biological Effects of Radiation*, Wykeham Pub. 1971.

Cole, Philip, et al, "Smoking and Cancer of Lower Urinary Tract," New Eng. J. of Med. 284:129-134, Jan. 21, 1971.

Day, Emerson, "Value of Regular Medical Examinations," Prevention of Cancer, pg. 366-70.

"Disease Control Programs – Cancer," U.S. Dept. HEW, Oct. 1966.

Doll, Sir Richard, "Smoking and Alcohol Together Hold Cause of Esophagus Cancer," Med. Tribune, Feb. 23, 1972.

Easson, E.C. and Russell, M.H., *The Curability of Cancer in Various Sites*, Williams & Wilkins, 1968.

"End Results in Cancer Report #3," U.S. Dept. HEW, 1968.

Gillespie, J.A., *Extracranial Cerebrovascular Disease and Its Management*, Bell & Bain Ltd., Glasgow, 1969.

Heath, C.W. Jr., "Clusters of Leukemia & Hodgkins Disease," New Eng. J. of Med., 284:129-134, Jan. 21, 1971.

Higgins, Ian, "The Epidemiology of Chronic Respiratory Disease," Prev. Med., Vol. 2, pg. 14-33, 1973.

Hilleman, M.R., "Vaccine for Marck's Disease in Chickens Seen as Big Advance," Med. Tribune, July 12, 1972.

Hilleman, M.R., "Cancer Vaccine is Foreseen Probably Only After Decades," Med. Tribune, Vol. 13, No. 8, Feb. 23, 1972.

Kannel, William, et al, "Left Ventricular Hypertrophy by Electrocardiogram Prevalence, Incidence and Mortality in the Framingham Study," Ann. Int. Med. 71:89-105, July 1969.

Kurtzke, J.F., *Epidemiology of Cerebrovascular Disease*, Springer-Verlag, 1969.

"Little Doubt of Virus-Ca Link; Vaccine Pursuit Held Practical," Medical Tribune, Jan. 9, 1974.

Lynch, H.T., *Hereditary Factors in Carcinoma*, Springer-Verlag Pub. 1967.

MacMahon, Brian, "Susceptibility to Radiation Induced Leukemia?," New Eng. J. of Med. 287:144-45, Sept. 20, 1972.

"Mortality from Cancer," Metropolitan Life Statistical Bulletin, Vol. 54, Feb. 1973.

"Mortality of Cerebrovascular Diseases," Metropolitan Life Statistical Bulletin, Vol. 54, Apr. 1973.

Moore, Condict, "Cigarette Smoking and Cancer of Mouth, Pharynx, and Larynx," JAMA 218:553-56.

"Patterns of Regional Longevity," Metropolitan Life Statistical Bulletin, Vol. 54, May 1973.

"Progress Against Cancer 1969," U.S. Dept. HEW, Nat. Adv. Council, U.S. Govt. Printing Office, Washington, D.C., 1969.

Prout, George Jr., "Current Concepts: Bladder Carcinoma," New Eng. J. of Med., 287:86-89, July 13, 1972.

Raven, Ronald W. & Roe, Francis J.C., *Prevention of Cancer*, Appleton, Century & Croft Pub. 1967.

"'Retirement May Militate Against Long Life," Med. Tribune, Jan. 23, 1974.

Schottenfeld, D., "Patient Risk Factors and Detection of Early Cancer," Prev. Med., Vol. 1, No. 3, pg. 335-51, Aug. 1972.

Silverberg, E. and Holleb, A., "Cancer Statistics 1972," Ca – A Cancer Jol. for Clinicians, Vol. 22, Jan./Feb. 1972.

Smillie, J.G., "Physician Questions Value of Annual Check Up" Am. Med. News, Jan. 17, 1972.

Smith Richard, "Possibilities and Problems of Immunologic Intervention in Cancer," New Eng. J. of Med. 287:439-450, Aug. 31, 1972.

Stuart, Marie J., et al, "Platelet Function in Recipients from Donors Ingesting Aspirin," New Eng. J. of Med., Vol. 287, No. 22, pg. 1105-08, Nov. 30, 1972.

Vital Statistics of the United States, *General Mortality*, Vol. II, Superintendant of Documents, 1967.

Wynder, Ernest L. et al, "The Epidemiology of Lung Cancer," JAMA, 213-2221-28, Sept. 28, 1970.

Wynder, E.L. & Mabuchi, K., "Gastrointestinal Cancer – Etiology And Environmental Factors," JAMA, Vol. 226, No. 13, pg. 1546-48, Dec. 24, 1973.

Wynder, E.L. & Mabuchi, K., "Lung Cancer Among Cigar and Pipe Smokers," Prev. Med., Vol. 1, pg. 529-542, Dec. 1972.

Zankel, Harry T., *Stroke Rehabilitation*, Chas. Thomas, 1971.

CHAPTERS XIV AND XV

Adult Decision Making Workshop #2, National Conf. on Smoking and Health, San Diego, Sept. 1970.

Fingerland, A., "Half of Infarction Deaths Linked to Smoking," Med. Tribune, Nov. 8, 1972.

Kiefer, N.C., "Accidents – The Foremost Problem in Preventive Medicine," Prev. Med., Vol. 2, 106-22, 1973.

"Mortality and Diabetes," Metropolitan Life Statistical Bulletin, Vol. 54, Dec. 1973.

Neel, J.V., *The Genetics of Diabetes Mellitus*, Acad. Press, 1970.

Rimoin, D.L. and Schemke, R. N., *Genetic Disorders of the Endocrine Glands*, C.V. Mosby Co. 1971.

Steinfield, J.L., "Technogenic Disease – The Price of Progress?," Prev. Med., Vol. 1:222-230, Mar. 1972.

Vital Statistics of the United States, *General Mortality*, Vol. II, Superintendant of Documents, 1967.

Index